THE
PALEO
THYROID
SOLUTION

ELLE RUSS

With in-depth commentary from
integrative physician Gary E. Foresman, MD

Library of Congress Control Number: 2016932163
Library of Congress Cataloging-in-Publication Data is on file with the publisher
Russ, Elle 1973-
Paleo Thyroid Solution/Elle Russ

ISBN: 978-1-939563-24-8
1. Thyroid Health 2. Diet 3. Weight loss

Design and Layout: Caroline De Vita
Illustrations: Caroline De Vita
Cover Design: Janée Meadows
Cover Photography and Professional Photo of Elle: Jonathan Moeller
Editor: Penelope Jackson
Consultant: Dr. Gary Forsman
Proofreader: Tim Tate
Index: Tim Tate
Other photos used by permission ©: iStock: 4maksym, bjonesmedia, brians101, Katrina Brown, cislander, dina2001, elenaleonova, Vitaly Edush, Christopher Futcher, Adrian Hillman, ivosar, Magone, mycola, rafal_olechowski, Rod Pforr, Ivelin Radkov, Alex Raths, Tverdohlib, Michael Utech, zeljkosantrac; **Shutterstock:** Shane Myers Photography, Dennis van de Water; **Dollar Photo Club:** kovalto1

Publisher: Primal Blueprint Publishing, 1641 S. Rose Ave., Oxnard, CA 93033
For information on quantity discounts, please call 888-774-6259,
email: info@primalblueprintpublishing.com,
or visit PrimalBlueprintPublishing.com.

TABLE OF CONTENTS

ACKNOWLEDGMENTS

I am filled with the utmost gratitude for
the man responsible for helping me change my life
and saving me from a future riddled with weight issues,
food addictions, adrenal problems,
suboptimal thyroid hormone metabolism,
and declining health.

Mark Sisson, *you are my* hero!

I suffered for a total of five years of my life due to undiagnosed hypo-thyroidism and Reverse T3 hypothyroidism. Unfortunately, my story is not unique, because like millions of thyroid patients, I was unable to find a doctor or an endocrinologist who was informed enough to fix my hypothyroidism. After two miserable years of being undiagnosed, I finally took my health into my own hands and became my own doctor. It was a scary place to be, feeling neglected by the medical community and the more than fifty highly regarded physicians I had spoken to. If I had trouble finding a doctor to help me in Los Angeles, I cannot even imagine how hard it would be to go through this ordeal in the smaller towns and cities throughout the United States.

When I decided to reject the dead-end mainstream medical journey I was on, my body and health were deteriorating so rapidly that I spent every day in full-blown misery, riddled with more than thirty hypothy-roid symptoms. Trying to start with a clean slate and be open to all pos-sibilities, I ordered my own lab work, bought thyroid hormones from assorted Internet resources without a prescription, and headed down a more holistic path to wellness. And it actually worked. It worked phe-nomenally well, for a while.

I was hit with a second bout of hypothyroidism in 2011 called Reverse T3—a once rare though increasingly common thyroid issue that many doctors have no idea how to test or fix. For the second time in ten years, I was on my own again, having to doctor myself back to health. Once again, I was successful.

Even though I am a writer (focused on TV and film—Hollywood stuff), I never had the intention of writing a thyroid book or anything health related. However, it seemed that everywhere I went I would run into someone suffering from hypothyroidism—either undiagnosed or unsuccessfully treated by their current doctor. We would somehow land on this topic without any prompting from me. After speaking with and offering help to over a hundred former strangers with thyroid issues, it began to feel like a calling. My close association with Mark Sisson and the Primal Blueprint movement made it clear to me that my calling is about integrating paleo/primal lifestyle methods to stimulate holistic healing of assorted thyroid conditions that, frankly, the medical community is failing to address through traditional means.

One of the worst symptoms of hypothyroidism is insidious weight gain and an inability to lose excess body fat, despite devoted efforts to hard workouts and restricting calories. After I was optimized on thyroid hormone replacement and over the challenge of my second bout of hypothyroidism, I tried every diet and lifestyle plan out there, to no avail. I started to believe a common and monumentally destructive misconception that some doctors pass on to their patients: "You have hypothyroidism, so you will always struggle with weight issues."

While it's true that even after people optimized on thyroid hormone replacement have eradicated 99.9% of their hypothyroid symptoms, they often just can't lose that excess weight without struggle, there is a solution.

And there is more to the Paleo Thyroid Solution than the ability to effortlessly lose stubborn excess weight. Adopting a paleo/primal lifestyle is the quickest and surest way to optimize thyroid hormone metabolism—for everyone with thyroid problems *and for everyone without thyroid problems*. Every human being has a thyroid gland, and as the master gland of the body, it plays a critical role in all metabolic processes. If thyroid hormone metabolism is not up to par, anyone one can be thrown down the spiral slide into a pool of weight gain and is at risk of developing an assortment of thyroid-related health problems.

Hypothyroidism, Hashimoto's disease, and Reverse T3 issues are on the rise. It is imperative that doctors who treat thyroid patients learn all they can about the latest treatment protocols in order to help their patients get well. In the meantime, I am overjoyed to present you with hope, encouragement, and a detailed plan to fix hypothyroidism. And if you're overwhelmed right now, if you're feeling lost and scared and unsure whether you'll ever make it through, please turn to chapter 8 and start with the stories of people who have been exactly where you are and found their way to health and happiness. Then meet me back at chapter 1 and we will start you on your own journey toward achieving vibrant health.

In **chapter 1** you will learn how the thyroid gland works and how it can malfunction.

In **chapter 2** you will learn about common symptoms and how to properly diagnose thyroid issues.

In **chapter 3** you will learn about applicable supplements and thyroid hormone replacement options, along with dosing strategies.

In **chapter 4** you will learn about the very uncommon protocol of T3-only dosing, along with a rarely discussed thyroid issue called Reverse T3.

In **chapter 5** you will learn about how paleo/primal food and exercise principles support vibrant health and thyroid hormone optimization and promote weight loss.

In **chapter 6** you will learn about your adrenal gland, and paleo/primal lifestyle principles and how they affect cortisol and glucose which have a major role in your thyroid health.

In **chapter 7** you will learn a stepwise approach to implementing the Paleo Thyroid Solution.

In **chapter 8** you'll read some Paleo Thyroid Solution success stories, including mine.

In **appendix I** is my captivating interview with integrative physician (and "primal doc") Gary E. Foresman, MD. I urge you to read it closely for insight into how and why doctors are getting things wrong and how thyroid health needs to be tested and treated.

In **appendix II** you will find my favorite paleo/primal resources along with other resources to help you on your healing journey.

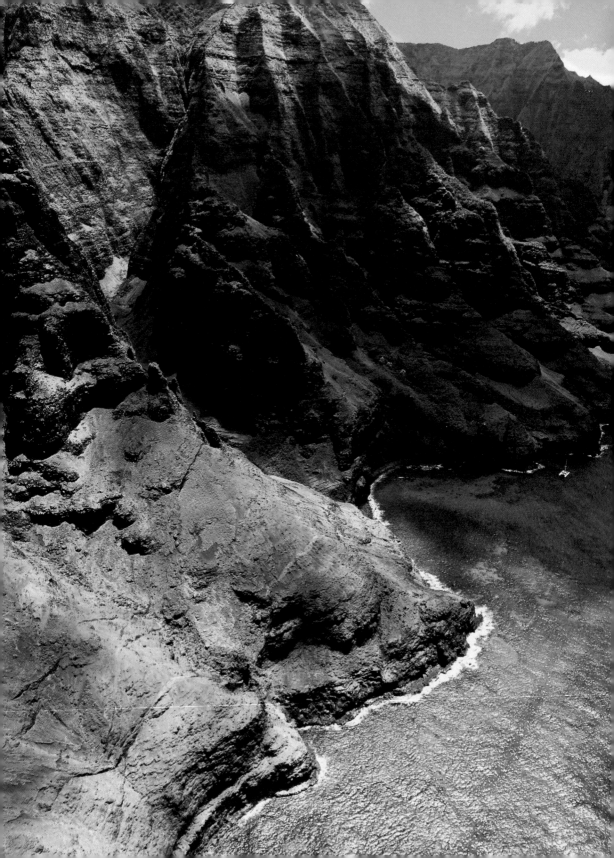

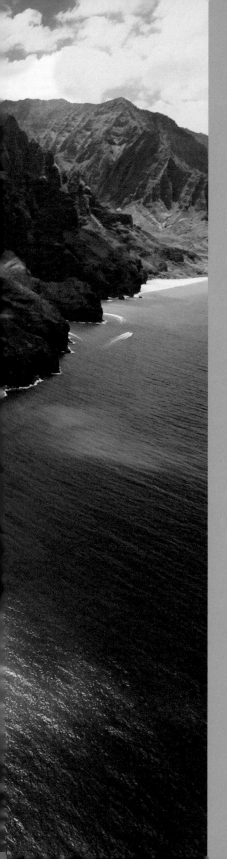

CHAPTER ONE

The Thyroid—Your Master Gland

Until now, you might not have paid attention to how the thyroid gland works or known about the critical role it plays in every aspect of physical health and mental well-being. Unfortunately, until a problem occurs and causes disease, the thyroid gland remains overlooked and misunderstood. This chapter offers an in-depth look at this miraculous tiny gland and what can go wrong with it.

The Thyroid Epidemic

There is a big discrepancy among experts' estimates of how many thyroid patients exist in the United States. The common assessment seems to be about 20 million Americans, while some groups estimate 27 million—with 13 million of them undiagnosed. Roughly 200 million people worldwide have some form of thyroid disease, and 60% of those with thyroid disease are undiagnosed and unaware of their condition. Undiagnosed hypothyroidism can put patients at risk for serious conditions, such as cardiovascular disease, high blood pressure, depression, osteoporosis, diabetes, infertility, and other gynecological disorders/hormone issues, and other diseases. More common in women, it is estimated that one in eight women will develop a thyroid disorder during her lifetime.

Hypothyroidism, an underactive thyroid disorder and the main subject of this book, is disproportionately a woman's disease. It's chronically misdiagnosed; doctors often mistake the symptoms of hypothyroidism as symptoms of other conditions, without factoring thyroid dysfunction as a potential *cause* of those symptoms. Instead, the patient is given a prescription for the misdiagnosed condition (such as high blood pressure or depression)—and the patient remains hypothyroid and continues to deteriorate. Even when properly diagnosed, hypothyroidism is often treated with the wrong combination and/or wrong dosage levels of thyroid hormones along with the widespread unavailability of proper nutritional coaching. Both the absence of treatment and the widespread practice of mistreatment results in unnecessary suffering while creating a platform of disease within the body that eventually leads to other life-threatening conditions, such as diabetes/metabolic syndrome, high blood pressure, depression, miscarriages, infertility, a variety of gynecological disorders, inflammation-related diseases, cancers, and more.

Twice in ten years, I struggled with hypothyroidism—I was slowly dying. As I mentioned in the introduction, I saw and corresponded with over fifty doctors during these two bouts, and no one knew how to help me either time. The reason all of those doctors failed to diagnose me is that they all ordered the same, incorrect blood tests, which is a widespread problem. (More on blood tests in chapter 2). I could feel my brain and body deteriorating rapidly, and I had developed a variety of other health problems caused by hypothyroidism and the low metabolic rate that goes hand in hand with it. It was frightening to say the least. If my thyroid condition continued to go unresolved longer than it had, I can only imagine the countless medical atrocities that would have ensued. I had already been *misdiagnosed* with another disease (PCOS, or Polycystic Ovary Syndrome); I developed a uterine fibroid and a uterine polyp (which later had to be surgically removed); and I had alarmingly low hormone and nutrient levels of all kinds. What else was in store for me? How many more health disasters would I have experienced before I met an extremely premature demise? How many more years of my life would be wasted on this disease? These are the thoughts that motivated me to write this book so I could help save others from the grim reality of undiagnosed and mistreated hypothyroidism.

The only way to prevent yourself from rapidly deteriorating from hypothyroidism or living a sub-par existence with sluggish thyroid function is to learn all that you can about the condition, become your own thyroid expert, and take control of your own health so that you can help yourself and your doctor treat it correctly. Had I known what I know now and could travel back in time, I would go back to my pre-hypothyroid days and immediately adopt a paleo lifestyle along with naturally optimizing certain hormone and nutrient levels in my body. Had I done that I might have avoided a life of being dependent on thyroid hormone replacement and I would have likely evaded the physical and mental tragedies of the slew of hypothyroid symptoms I suffered from. Before we detail the amazing way I have found to solve my thyroid issues, let's explore just what this little gland does.

Your Thyroid—The Master Gland

All vertebrates have a thyroid gland: humans, mammals, birds, reptiles, amphibians, and fishes. The thyroid is a butterfly-shaped gland located on the front of and in the middle of your neck.

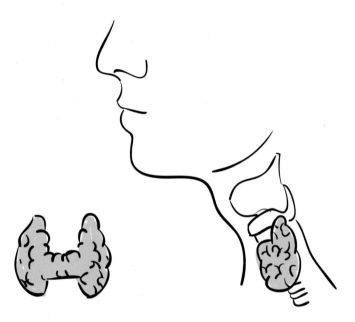

You cannot live without a thyroid gland. Well, technically you can live without the actual gland, but you must give your body what the missing thyroid gland once gave you: thyroid hormones. The reason you cannot stay alive without a thyroid gland—or, more importantly, *adequate levels of thyroid hormones*—is that the thyroid is the master gland of the human body. The thyroid gland controls the metabolic rate of every organ in the body, from the production and regulation of sex hormones, adrenal hormones, body temperature, growth development, brain function, and heart rate, to every other element that keeps your body functioning. Inadequate thyroid hormones in the human body will ultimately contribute to a miserable existence, likely rampant with diseases and health problems.

WHAT IS METABOLIC RATE?

Metabolic rate involves the entire range of biological processes that occur within us. It involves the *buildup* and *breakdown* of substances—most often used to describe the breakdown of food and its transformation into energy. Your body can use the fuel for energy, or store the energy in body tissues like your muscles, liver, and body fat.

In cases where a person has their thyroid surgically removed, they are given thyroid hormone replacement in order to live. If that same person were stranded on an island with a supply of food but had no thyroid hormones available, they would have difficulty surviving, because thyroid hormones control the metabolic rate for every single organ in the body—and in their absence the body will continue to deteriorate rapidly.

"Thyroid function is very complex and exerts a profound effect on the function of nearly every other organ in the body. Therefore, smooth functioning of the overall body chemistry depends on the health of your thyroid gland."
—Christiane Northrup, MD, drnorthrup.com

Adopting a paleo/primal lifestyle positively affects thyroid hormone metabolism more than any other way of eating and more than any other lifestyle strategy. This applies to people who currently don't have thyroid issues and to people who take thyroid hormone replacement. In order to achieve optimal thyroid hormone metabolism, living a paleo existence is a great path for people who want to recover from hypothyroidism naturally or seek to optimize their current thyroid hormone replacement. You'll get all the details you need on the paleo approach to health and vitality in chapter 6.

The Midwest "Goiter Belt"

The Midwest is sometimes referred to as the "Goiter Belt." A goiter is an enlarged thyroid gland caused by inadequate iodine, which aggravates the thyroid as it tries to keep up with thyroid hormone production. A goiter can grow larger than the size of a cantaloupe.

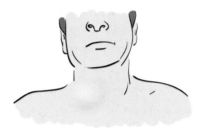

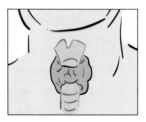
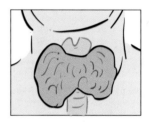

This inland region of the United States that surrounds the Great Lakes used to be a hotbed of goiter activity back in the day, the cause of which was thought to be a diet based on foods grown in iodine-depleted soil. As a response, iodized salt was introduced to the diet, and it successfully eliminated the Goiter Belt in the Midwest and other select areas of the country. Iodine deficiency was the most common cause of thyroid goiters.

How The Thyroid Gland Works

The thyroid gland gets activated to release thyroid hormones into the bloodstream via a signal sent from the pituitary gland at the base of our brains called the TSH (Thyroid Stimulating Hormone). (Side note: TSH is neither a thyroid hormone nor an accurate blood test to use alone in assessing thyroid health—a common practice of uninformed doctors). TSH is a pituitary hormone and TSH levels only indicate to us how loud or soft the signal being sent to the thyroid is. What truly matters is how the thyroid gland *interprets that TSH signal*…meaning whether or not the thyroid gland dispenses enough thyroid hormones to the body after receiving the TSH signal. Furthermore, even if the thyroid gland releases hormones into the body, those hormones need to get metabolized properly in the body or the person will remain hypothyroid. Sometimes, the pituitary doesn't send the TSH signal at all.

The Main Hormones—T4 & T3

The two main thyroid hormones the thyroid releases are T4 (thyroxine) and T3 (triiodothyronine). These are the only ones measurable via blood tests and the only ones to be concerned with when it comes to thyroid health. Approximately 80% of T4 is released by the thyroid. Approximately 7–20% of T3 is released by the thyroid.

T4 is a prohormone, and its job is to *convert into the biologically active thyroid hormone T3*. T3 is the *fuel and energy that keeps us alive* (more on T3 in a bit). When the pituitary senses a lack of T4 and T3 in the blood, it sends the TSH signal to the thyroid to produce more thyroid hormones. As we'll see, sometimes the thyroid doesn't take the bait. Or, it takes the bait but only releases suboptimal amounts of thyroid hormones.

FOUR PROCESSES OF FAT-BURNING METABOLISM

1. The thyroid gland outputting T4 and T3
   (or you taking thyroid hormone replacement)
2. Your body converts the T4 into T3
3. The T3 arriving at work (the cells)
4. The T3 "punching in" to work (enter/affects the cells)

Why doesn't the thyroid gland just pump T3 directly into our system, if that's what our bodies ultimately need? Why does the thyroid bother with this "middleman" T4 and this whole conversion process? T3 is the biologically active, most important thyroid hormone to human health, and as a result, it's a very powerful energy hormone. T3 has such immediate and powerful effects that our bodies sort of have a built-in time-release process, where T3 is wisely dispensed to our bodies via T4 throughout the day when our bodies need it. The biologically inactive T4 converts into the biologically active T3. The leftover T4 that was not converted into T3 will convert, instead, into a biologically inactive form of T3 called Reverse T3 (RT3), as a way of clearing out excess T4 from the body that goes unused/unconverted.

T3 THYROID FUNCTION—THE HORMONE OF LIFE

There is really only *one* thyroid hormone that we know for a fact is critical to life, and that hormone is called T3 (triiodothyronine). T3 is extremely powerful and is responsible for fat burning, brain function, body temperature, healthy heart rate, healthy blood pressure, physical energy, and more. T3 *is* energy. Having adequate levels of T3 contributes to lean muscle mass and calorie burning. T3 is what keeps your body temperature at an average of 98.6°F in healthy humans.

T3 is so powerful that your body has an extremely smart mechanism in place that protects you from the energy effects of T3 by dishing it out to your bloodstream incrementally via the other thyroid hormone T4. The thyroid gland releases some T3 directly into the bloodstream, but 80% of what the thyroid releases is T4. The job of the T4, either released from your thyroid gland or ingested as thyroid hormone replacement, is to convert into life-giving T3. We cannot live without T3, and very low or inadequate levels of T3 in our system will negatively affect other biological systems.

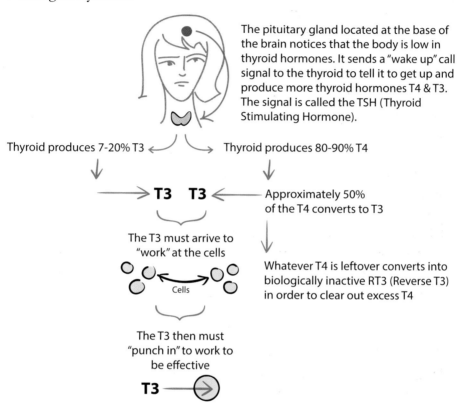

The pituitary gland located at the base of the brain notices that the body is low in thyroid hormones. It sends a "wake up" call signal to the thyroid to tell it to get up and produce more thyroid hormones T4 & T3. The signal is called the TSH (Thyroid Stimulating Hormone).

Thyroid produces 7-20% T3

Thyroid produces 80-90% T4

T3   T3 ← Approximately 50% of the T4 converts to T3

The T3 must arrive to "work" at the cells

Cells

Whatever T4 is leftover converts into biologically inactive RT3 (Reverse T3) in order to clear out excess T4

The T3 then must "punch in" to work to be effective

T3 ⟶

THYROID HORMONE FUNCTION

On a daily basis, the thyroid gland releases: **T4, T3, T2, T1 & calcitonin**.

- **T4**: 80–93% of what your thyroid produces. Its main function is to convert into the biologically active hormone T3. Of the T4 produced by the thyroid gland, 40–50% converts into T3.
- **T3**: 7–20% of total production by thyroid. Most of the T3 in your body makes its appearance when T4 loses one of its molecules to become T3—a peripheral (that is, away from thyroid gland) conversion of T4 to T3 in the body.

- **T2**: May play a role in production of an enzyme called deiodinase that helps covert T4 to T3.
- **T1**: May play a role in keeping thyroid function in check.
- **Calcitonin**: Primarily secreted by thyroid, calcitonin responds to too-high levels of calcium in the blood and inhibits the release of more calcium from your bones to the blood.

T4, T3 AND REVERSE T3—THE MAIN ATTRACTIONS

There is currently no compelling scientific evidence that suggests T1, T2, and calcitonin are necessary for longevity and optimal thyroid hormone metabolism. Many successful thyroid hormone replacement options have zero T1, T2, or calcitonin in them, and people live long, healthy lives without these extra thyroid hormones.

The ultimate goal of the thyroid gland is to get your body enough T4 so it will convert into adequate levels of T3 in order to keep you alive and well (at the same time, our thyroid gives us some direct T3 as well). *For T4 to be useful at all, it must convert into T3.* There is no scientific evidence at this time that suggests T4 itself is necessary to longevity or healthy thyroid hormone metabolism. Adequate T3 levels and thyroid hormone metabolism are the ultimate goals when it comes to thyroid health. As an example, people who are on T3-only thyroid hormone replacement like myself, have had no T4 in their system for years, and we live vibrantly healthy lives.

T4 IS WORTHLESS UNLESS IT TURNS INTO T3

T4 to T3 conversion primarily happens within the cells of the thyroid, liver, kidneys, some in the gut, and through the action of a specific enzyme called the D1 deiodinase. A small portion of the conversion from T4 to T3 happens within the gastrointestinal tract, but only if the gut is healthy and has the right level of friendly gut bacteria. Some conversion also occurs within the cells of the brain, bones, muscles, through the action of another specific enzyme called the D2 deiodinase. The mineral selenium also plays a key role in the conversion of T4 to T3. Whatever remaining T4 has not converted into T3 will be converted into the *biologically inactive* Reverse T3 (RT3) in order to clear out the excess T4.

If, for any reason, the T4 that is released by your thyroid gland (or taken orally) does not convert into the biologically active T3, but instead converts into RT3, you will experience hypothyroid symptoms, the severity of which depends on how little T4 is being converted into T3 along with how well the T3 is affecting the cells (more on Reverse T3 in chapter 4).

T3 IS USELESS UNTIL IT "PUNCHES IN" TO WORK

Imagine that the cells are the office building, and the punch card machine is inside the building. T3 must arrive at the cells and then "punch in" to the cells in order to be effective. Having T3 merely circulating in your bloodstream is not enough to guarantee health and eliminate hypothyroid symptoms. In fact, if T3 is just circulating in your bloodstream and not getting into the cells to act in them, T3 will remain useless. When someone has a Reverse T3 problem (that's when the T4 converts into the biologically *inactive* form of T3), what happens is the T3 sort of just floats around in the bloodstream, inactive, like water contained in a pool, not going anywhere. In this case, T3 does not go into the office building—and does not punch in to work (and therefore cannot affect the cells). You can think about Reverse T3 like a blockade or a locked door preventing T3 from doing its job. There are a few ways to go about correcting Reverse T3 issues, which we'll explore in chapter 4.

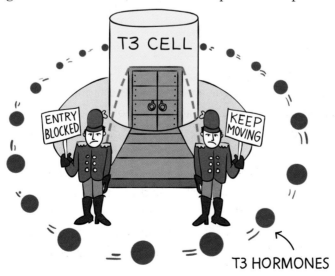

T4 to T3 Conversion Issues

Your own thyroid may be dispensing enough T4, or a hypothyroid patient can ingest T4, but if that T4 is not converting properly into the biologically active hormone T3, then T4 is useless and it will ultimately be harmful to the patient, because they will become hypothyroid. There are a variety of factors that can cause T4 to T3 conversion issues, such as a sluggish or unhealthy liver, poor diet, adrenal dysfunction, vitamin/mineral deficiencies, low iron storage, and blood sugar imbalances. Chronic dieting, overexercising, and caloric restriction can affect T4 to T3 conversion because your body thinks it's starving, so it slows down thyroid hormone production to prevent your body from burning any more fat. Doing chronic cardio (a pattern of frequent workouts where you exceed 75% of your max heart rate for a sustained period of time) can negatively affect thyroid hormone metabolism by skewing the output and balance of adrenal hormones and glucose metabolism, both of which are connected to thyroid health.

Hypothyroidism generally stems from one (or more) of these categories:

1. The pituitary gland does not produce enough TSH.
2. The thyroid gland does not release enough T4 and T3 in response to the TSH.
3. T4 is not converting into enough T3.
4. T4 is converting into the inactive Reverse T3.
5. Hashimoto's disease is an autoimmune disease whereby the immune system creates antibodies that attack the thyroid gland (attempting to destroy it). Sometimes a combination of both hypothyroidism and hyperthyroidism can occur.

Hyperthyroidism generally stems from:

1. Graves' disease is an autoimmune disease whereby the immune system creates antibodies (proteins produced by the body to protect against a virus or bacteria) called thyroid-stimulating immunoglobulin (TSI).

These antibodies turn on the thyroid and cause it to grow and secrete more thyroid hormones than your body needs. This is by far the most common cause of hyperthyroidism.

2. *Excessive thyroid hormones produced for other reasons, such as nodules in the thyroid gland or too much iodine.*

3. *Ingesting too high a dosage of thyroid replacement hormones.*

Human Kryptonite

The true kryptonite of the human species is anything *anti-thyroid*. These are external influences such as food glutens, environmental chemicals (chlorine, bromine, fluoride), certain medications, soybeans and soy products, nuclear radiation, and even adverse health practices like too much stress, overexercising, poor diet, nutrient deficiencies, adrenal imbalances, blood sugar instability, and not enough sleep—all of which can throw off the delicate hormonal interactions that support optimal thyroid function and metabolism.

If humans will die without a thyroid gland (and zero thyroid hormones) what do you think will happen to someone who has long-term sluggish or suboptimal levels of thyroid hormones? Unresolved or untreated hypothyroidism can lead to a myriad of medical problems, including depression, insulin resistance and type 2 diabetes, blood pressure issues, cholesterol issues, gynecological issues, cancers, heart disease, infertility, and more.

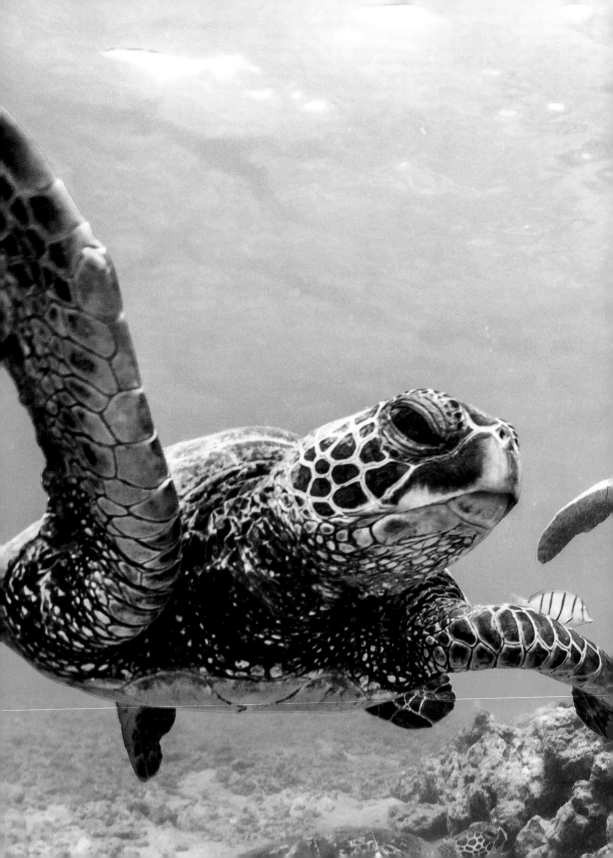

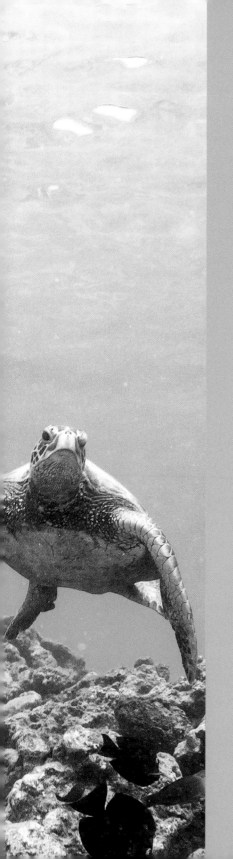

CHAPTER TWO

Symptoms, Causes, and Diagnosis of Hypothyroidism

*Life is great when the thyroid gland
is working properly, but when things
go haywire, it can affect every aspect
of your mind and body.
You might experience depression,
weight gain, lack of energy,
or perpetually cold hands and feet.
In this chapter we will explore
the consequences of unhealthy
thyroid function and how you can
get to the bottom of it.*

Hypothyroidism (and Reverse T3 Hypothyroidism) Symptoms

Trying to impart how it feels to experience full-blown hypothyroidism and its symptoms is akin to a woman attempting to explain menstrual cramps to a man; unless you have experienced it yourself, you cannot relate or understand. I had all but three or four symptoms on this list. Many hypothyroid symptoms are not visible to others, and oftentimes doctors and family members/friends think these symptoms are in one's head, somehow fabricated by a hypochondriac human mind. These symptoms are not only real, they are rampant in people suffering from undiagnosed or mistreated hypothyroidism.

- Cold hands/feet and generally being cold regardless of the weather or temperature
- Insidious weight gain
- Inability to lose weight no matter what you do
- Weak arms (Can be general weakness like not being able to hold something heavy for a long time and/or this might manifest as tendonitis or carpal tunnel syndrome.)
- Low energy and stamina
- Serious depression or general malaise (Aside from sadness and despair, hypo-depression sometimes manifests as the feeling of being *paralyzed with lack of motivation* and being unable to do anything about it, even though you know something is wrong with you. It's like you just can't seem to take action to help yourself.)
- *Needing* a nap every day
- Constipation
- Sluggish reflexes (I became very clumsy and would knock over everything and bump into everything, even though I am an extremely coordinated person in general.)
- Dry cracked skin (On heels, ankles, and sometimes it shows up on the inside edge of an index finger and looks like very dry, scaly, cracked skin.)
- Hair feels like a rubber band when touched or pulled (Yet it breaks easily.)

- Hair loss
- Loss of curliness in curly or wavy hair
- Inability to focus and concentrate (Extremely difficult to read, learn, or sustain mental focus, even while watching a film or a TV show. One has to reread paragraphs in order to retain the information. Someone could be talking to you and you can barely understand what they are saying and/or you instantly forget what they just said.)
- Mixing up words in speech (sort of like *dyslexia of the mouth*) and difficulty remembering words (Not being able to speak properly or get the words out correctly.)
- Lower/deeper voice or scratchy/raspy voice
- Brain fog and forgetfulness
- Menstrual irregularities such as heavy bleeding, constant bleeding, uterine fibroids/polyps, polycystic ovary syndrome (PCOS), miserable and long-lasting PMS
- Fibrocystic breasts (One or both breasts can be painful, sensitive, sore, achy, lumpy, which can also be a sign of estrogen dominance.)
- Infertility and miscarriages
- Weak, brittle, cracking, breaking, splitting fingernails
- Achy muscles and overall soreness
- Blood pressure issues (high or low)
- Itchy inner ears (It's like trying to scratch an itch that you cannot reach, even with a cotton swab. This one drove me nuts!)
- Heavy legs when walking (feels like you are walking with cement legs)
- Unhealthy cholesterol results
- Low body temperature (details on page 86)
- Uncomfortable feeling in the throat/neck area (Feeling "choked up," similar to when you are about to cry or when you feel like you can't speak in a stressful situation, that "lump in your throat" feeling. Difficulty swallowing, constantly clearing one's throat, and/or not wanting clothing to cover or touch the neck.)
- Digestive problems (gas, abdominal bloating)

- Problems at work or the inability to function well at work
- Relationship issues with family/friends, romantic partners, and/or colleagues, etc.
- Increased or uncontrollable cravings for sugar and carbohydrates
- Allergies (rare allergies are often related to untreated or mis-treated Hashimoto's)
- Messy handwriting (Issues with brain-hand-muscle dexterity can lead to messy handwriting; it feels hard to get the words from your brain through your hand onto the paper.)
- Heart palpitations (Especially when lying down, it feels as though your heart is pumping and thumping loud and strong in your chest and you are "aware" of your heartbeat like never before, and it feels scary. Often related to adrenals and/or low iron.)
- Restless legs, uncontrollable compulsion to continually readjust one's legs (Feels like you cannot find a comfortable position for your legs. Especially annoying at night while trying to sleep. Often related to low iron.)
- Compromised immunity (Getting colds and/or flus more often than before.)
- Extended recovery needed after exercise and sore after exercise
- Sensitivity to light, sounds, and smells (Often related to adrenals.)
- Low or zero sex drive
- Moody, sensitive, easily agitated, and feeling overwhelmed by simple everyday tasks (Just thinking about doing a load of laundry can feel overwhelming/stressful and bring a hypothyroid person to tears.)
- Swelling and inflammation
- Puffy eyes and face upon waking, and a general feeling of overall puffiness and bloat
- Myxedema (Swelling of the skin and underlying tissues is typical of patients with underactive thyroid glands. Discoverable by visual assessment and not being able to pinch a miniscule bit of skin on the outside of your arms, near your shoulders. *Instead* one is only able to pinch a thick, large portion of skin.)

- Stomach fat and a growing "tire" around your waist (thyroid *and* adrenal related)
- Headaches
- Constant thirst and water won't quench it
- Feeling as if something wrong is happening to your brain, as if you are getting "dumb" and losing your cognitive abilities
- Anxiety attacks

Hashimoto's Symptoms

The demolition of the thyroid gland, which is caused by the immune system attacking it, can cause patients to feel hypothyroid one day and hyperthyroid another day. All of the hypothyroid symptoms can apply to Hashimoto's, and the following list of hyperthyroid symptoms might also apply.

- Easily fatigued
- Depression
- Dry skin and hair (and eyes)
- Lower body temperature, feeling cold
- Unexplainable weight gain
- Constipation
- Serious discomfort in the neck/throat area

Hyperthyroid Symptoms

- Increased bowel movements, with or without diarrhea
- Weight loss, inability to gain weight
- Agitation, aggressiveness, impatience
- Anxiety, panic attacks
- Shakiness or jitteriness
- Insomnia or difficulties sleeping
- Rapid heartbeat, chest pain, heart palpitations
- Less frequent or irregular menstrual periods
- Inability to remain still, constantly fidgeting

- Throat tightness
- Thyroid nodules
- Increased sweating and feeling warmer than most people around you
- Sensitivity/intolerance to heat
- Increased appetite
- Goiter
- Prominent, bulging eyes or "bug eyes"
- Inflammation
- Irritability
- Dry eyes and gritty, sandpaper-like feeling in the eyes when you blink or close them (Feels like you need to use eye drops several times a day.)
- Muscle weakness
- Shortness of breath (Sometimes detectable after walking uphill or up a flight of stairs and feeling more winded and exhausted than one should for the exertion.)

Potential Causes of Hypothyroidism

If you have any of these conditions or lifestyle habits, it's important to be aware of how they can affect your thyroid function. Be vigilant in taking care of your own health.

- Selenium deficiency
- Iron deficiency
- Starvation
- Dieting
- Overexercising
- Adrenal issues/stress (low and/or high cortisol)
- Reverse T3 (T4 to T3 conversion issues)
- Hashimoto's (Can be triggered by the consumption of grains/gluten.)
- Congenital hypothyroidism, or hypothyroidism present at birth
- Surgical removal of part, or all of the thyroid gland

- Radiation treatment of the thyroid gland
- Pituitary gland abnormalities (rare)
- Emotional/mental causes
- Carbohydrate dependency/sugar addiction
- Diabetes

Diagnosing Hypothyroidism

There are three main methods of diagnosing hypothyroidism and using all three can accurately assess thyroid issues: tracking symptoms, measuring body temperature, and blood tests.

SYMPTOMS

The amount, variety, and severity of hypothyroid symptoms that people experience are highly individual and based on how low your levels of T3 are in your body. (Or in the case of hyperthyroidism, how abnormally *elevated* your T3 levels are.) If you have been treated for hypothyroidism but are still experiencing any of the hypothyroid symptoms mentioned, it is likely that you are either not on the right dosage of thyroid hormone replacement and/or you are having issues with T4 to T3 conversion (more on this in chapter 4.).

BODY TEMPERATURE

Humans should have an average afternoon body temperature of 98.6°F. Although our bodies go through fluctuations in temperature throughout the day based on activity, illness, weather, etc., the internal thermostat for humans is set at 98.6°F.

- Normal basal body temperature range (immediately upon waking) should be between 97.8°F and 98.2°F.
- Healthy mid-afternoon body temperature (around 3:00 p.m.) is 98.6°F.

Many hypothyroid sufferers have a *lower* than normal body temperature (below 97.8°F as a basal temperature and below 98.6°F in the afternoon). Hyperthyroid sufferers have *higher* than normal temperature (basal temperature consistently at top of basal range 98.2°F/98.3°F and an afternoon temperature consistently above 98.6°F). When I was seriously hypothyroid, my body temperature was 96°F on most days and never reached 98.6°F until I was optimized on thyroid hormone replacement. When I was hyperthyroid, my basal temperature was around 98.3°F and my afternoon temperature was 99°F.

Not only can assessing body temperature help with diagnosing hypothyroidism, it can also be used to gauge whether or not you are on the optimal dosage of thyroid hormone replacement (i.e., if you have been on thyroid hormones for a while but your afternoon temperature never reaches 98.5°/98.6°F, you might need more thyroid hormones).

Test your BASAL body temperature:
1. Get one of the following: an old-school mercury thermometer or a Geratherm thermometer. (Geratherm is an alternative to the mercury thermometers—digital thermometers are not as reliable.)
2. Place thermometer within arm's reach of your bed.
3. Upon waking in the morning, *before sitting up or leaving your bed*, put the thermometer under your tongue and relax for seven to ten minutes. Yes, this is a long time, but it will ensure an accurate temperature reading.
4. Remove the thermometer and record your temperature.

Test your MID-AFTERNOON body temperature (around 3:00 pm):
1. Get one of the following: an old-school mercury thermometer or a Geratherm thermometer.
2. Sit quietly for at least fifteen minutes before taking your temperature.
3. Don't eat, drink, smoke, or exercise, during this time.
4. Sit comfortably and put the thermometer under your tongue for a solid seven to ten minutes.
5. Remove the thermometer and record your temperature.

If your basal temperature is consistently below 97.8°F and/or your mid-afternoon temperature is consistently below 98.6°F:

- It's indicative of hypothyroidism.
- If you are already on thyroid hormone replacement, you may not be on the right dosage, the right type/combination of thyroid hormones, or the T4 is not converting into T3 (Reverse T3).
- Wacky adrenals, low iron, and/or poor food choices are issues keeping you hypothyroid.

If your basal temperature is consistently 98.2°/98.3°F or *above* and/or your mid-afternoon temperature is *above* 98.6°F:

- Your thyroid gland could be dispensing too much thyroid hormone (hyperthyroidism).
- You might be on too much thyroid hormone replacement, which is causing you to be hyperthyroid.
- You might have low iron, low aldosterone, or low estrogen.
- Adrenal issues: you might be producing too much adrenaline (manifests as anxiety attacks, feeling jittery/shaky, and/or heart palpitations).

Blood Tests—What to Look for and What Gets Missed

In my experience, every time hypothyroidism goes unnoticed by a doctor, it is usually because they are not ordering the correct blood tests and/or they are misinterpreting blood tests. During my first bout of hypothyroidism, I went undiagnosed for two years by a slew of doctors who only ordered the TSH test. TSH is the most *inaccurate* way of assessing thyroid health, and to this day, it remains the false standard for assessing thyroid problems.

RECOMMENDED THYROID TESTS

- Free T3
- Free T4

- TSH (This is not a test your doctor should rely on as a sole measurement in assessing hypothyroidism; nor should a doctor use this test on its own to prescribe or alter doses of T4, NDT, T4/T3 combination, or T3-only.)
- TPOAb (thyroid peroxidase antibody for Hashimoto's detection)
- TgAb (thyroglobulin antibody for Hashimoto's detection)
- Reverse T3 (must be taken in the same blood draw as Free T3)

RECOMMENDED THYROID-RELATED TESTS
- Vitamin D, 25-hydroxy
- Homocysteine
- B12
- Ferritin
- DHEA-sulfate
- Morning cortisol or twenty-four-hour saliva cortisol test
- Sex hormones for both sexes: free testosterone, progesterone, estradiol

Hypothyroidism throws off the balance of sex hormones and can also deplete them. You can test your sex hormones to see what your levels are, but just know that getting your thyroid gland working properly or getting optimized on the right dose of thyroid hormone replacement can correct the balance of sex hormones in the body (it did for me). As a result, I recommend you attempt thyroid hormone optimization *first*, before attempting sex hormone replacement.

Blood Lab Values
What is meant by "Free" T4 and T3? Free means unbound and circulating in your blood—and *available*. Here is what the Free T4, Free T3, and all of the other thyroid blood tests should look like.

If you're not used to looking at lab results, here are some things you should know. Every lab has its own normal range, which varies slightly from that of other labs. Some common lab ranges and corresponding results are presented below. And labs often measure using different units, so sometimes results are measured in picograms (one trillionth of a gram) per milliliter and sometimes they're measured in nanograms (one billionth of a gram) per deciliter. To avoid confusion, I eliminated the units of measurement in the blood tests in the results in this book, because the units of measure only matter if you're doing ratio calculations for Reverse T3, and you can choose those automatically on online Reverse T3 calculators. Otherwise, all you need to know is where your results fit within the lab's ranges.

FREE T4 (THYROXINE) AND FREE T3 (TRIIODOTHYRONINE)

Although individual, many people who are optimized on thyroid hormones *containing T3* will see the following themes in blood results (descriptions of hormone replacement options in chapter 3):

- A Free T4 around mid-range (usually 1.4 on standard test ranges)
- A Free T3 above mid-range, at the very top of the range, and sometimes a little over the range

Although lab reference ranges vary, the ranges following are commonly used. Whatever lab you use for your blood tests, if their reference ranges vary slightly from the ones shown here, it's easy to calculate what the middle of the range is.

FREE T3 LAB RESULTS

Free T3 lab range = (2.30–4.20)
Free T3 mid-range result = 3.0–3.3
Free T3 top-range result = 3.9–4.2

FREE T4 LAB RESULTS

Free T4 lab range = (0.82–1.77)
Free T4 mid-range result = 1.4
Free T4 top-range result = 1.6–1.77

OTHER FREE T4 AND FREE T3 LAB RESULT CONSIDERATIONS

- T3-only patients who are optimized sometimes have a Free T3 value of 10–20% over the range and a very low or non-existent Free T4 (a result such as <0.11).
- A low Free T4 can indicate hypothyroidism or a Reverse T3 problem (except in people taking T3-only).
- A high Free T4 can indicate hyperthyroidism.
- A high Free T4 combined with a high Free T3 can indicate a Reverse T3 problem.

Normal, Classic Blood Test Results in People with No Thyroid Issues

Below are the thyroid blood test results of a 44-year-old male with no thyroid symptoms or issues. This person lives a paleo/primal lifestyle and has a slim/trim physique with no hypothyroid symptoms whatsoever. His thyroid results are reflective of those who have normal, efficient thyroid hormone function.

TEST	RESULT	RANGE	NOTES
Free T3	3.2	(2.0–4.4)	mid-range and normal
Free T4	1.31	(0.82–1.77)	value 1.31 is classically normal
TSH	2.070	(0.450–4.500)	about mid-range (But TSH fluctuates so much that in the absence of Free T4 and Free T3 results, this test won't tell a complete story.)
Reverse T3	12.1	(9.2–24.1)	
Calculated RT3 Ratio: 26.4		over 20 is considered healthy	

Why Are So Many People Undiagnosed—And Why Are Patients Mistreated After Diagnosis?

- *Doctors sometimes treat a patient's symptoms without investigating **why** the symptoms appeared in the first place and what might be the **cause** of the symptoms. As a result, doctors can misdiagnose various symptoms of hypothyroidism as other conditions, such as depression, high blood pressure, high cholesterol, infertility, PCOS, bipolar disorder, sex hormone imbalance or deficiency.*

- *Some doctors have relied on and use outdated, irrelevant thyroid blood tests.*

- *Some doctors have relied strictly on lab reference ranges and test results.*

- *The medical community has failed to understand (and thus adequately treat) the synergistic connections between thyroid hormone levels and other processes in the body, such as the adrenal glands, blood glucose management, and nutrient levels like iron storage.*

- *Doctors can misunderstand T3 and subsequently be unnecessarily cautious in prescribing this hormone.*

- *Some doctors have failed to research and educate themselves on medical topics beyond what they learned in medical school. As a result, an alarming number of doctors and endocrinologists are not up to date with the latest thyroid treatments.*

- *Some doctors fail to administer optimal levels of thyroid hormones.*

- *Many doctors have adhered to flawed, conventional once-a-day thyroid hormone dosing for patients taking T3-containing hormone replacement.*

- *Big Pharma influence—money and business—has negatively affected hypothyroid patients for over fifty years due to its propaganda campaigns starting in the 1950s and continuing onward, touting T4-only treatment as a one-size-fits-all solution while simultaneously dispensing false information about NDT (natural desiccated thyroid) treatment.*

- *The medical community has failed to understand the connection between nutrition and thyroid health. As a result, doctors are unable to help hypothyroid patients reach optimal thyroid hormone metabolism*

A Word about Uninformed Doctors' Blind Reliance on Blood Test Values

Too many doctors and endocrinologists look for a patient's Free T3 to be in the middle of the range, and they are usually not flexible when it comes to labs results, because they are following old, outdated, conventional thyroid wisdom by looking for a specific number in the range. So if a lab result is higher in the range than the target number they are expecting, the doctor will reduce medication accordingly, which can keep people hypothyroid. They will also not take symptoms into account, so for example, someone's Free T3 might be where an endocrinologist might want it to be, but the patient is still complaining of hypothyroid symptoms. This endocrinologist will just make decisions according to the labs and ignore the individual patient. In my experience, seeing an endocrinologist for your thyroid health can seriously put you at risk for remaining hypothyroid due to rampant incorrect blood test assessment and widespread mistreatment fostered by reliance on T4-only hormone replacement. Having a Free T3 in the middle of the range doesn't work for everyone, including myself. Some people need to be high in the range, or even over the range (as long as hyperthyroid symptoms are not present). The American Association of Clinical Endocrinologists (AACE) guides endocrinologists to aim for a Free T3 in the middle of the range for their patients. (If they even test Free T3, which many do not.) This is extremely misguided, not only because every person's hormone needs are individual, but also they are basing this value on what "normal" people's thyroid tests look like.

Many uninformed doctors will say that because a patient's Free T3 is over the range on a blood test, it means that the patient is hyperthyroid, *which is flat out wrong.* Having a Free T3 *substantially over the range* might be a red flag, but having a Free T3 just a bit over the top of the range does not mean the patient is hyperthyroid! A patient is not hyperthyroid unless they exhibit hyperthyroid/overstimulation symptoms as listed earlier in this chapter. Overstimulation symptoms reveal themselves when someone is hyperthyroid; hyperthyroidism isn't a "sneaky condition" that hides itself only to be revealed by blood tests. Hyperthyroidism makes itself known through symptoms and vitals. *Vitals are measurable: body temperature, blood pressure, and heart rate.* Hyperthyroidism is *very noticeable and very uncomfortable* (I experienced it myself).

All too often, patients are kept hypothyroid and sick because their doctors overreact if they see their Free T3 result toward the top of the range or over the range. Unfortunately, without even attempting to see if overstimulation symptoms are present, the doctor may automatically reduce the patient's thyroid hormone dosage due to an unfounded fear that the patient has become hyperthyroid (based solely on blood work). Instead, doctors need to pay attention to measurable vitals and symptoms before assuming that a patient is hyperthyroid.

Thyroid-Stimulating Hormone—A *Pituitary* Hormone

Remember, the pituitary gland is responsible for sending wake-up calls to the thyroid gland to release thyroid hormones into the body through a signal called the TSH. In essence, the pituitary gland is an alarm clock for the thyroid, and sometimes the thyroid presses the snooze button when the alarm goes off, or never even gets out of bed. In some cases, the pituitary gland never sends the signal in the first place or doesn't release a strong enough signal to give a loud enough wake-up call for the thyroid to hear. When the thyroid does not produce adequate thyroid hormones for whatever reasons, the body enters a hypothyroid state. Even though testing a person's TSH is a common practice, TSH is *not a thyroid hormone* it is a *pituitary hormone.* The TSH blood test as a stand-alone thyroid test is an outdated, extremely ineffective way to gauge thyroid hormone metabolism (although it can assist with a diagnosis in the presence of both Free T4 and Free T3 lab results).

The validity of TSH is akin to placing an order with an online store. It doesn't matter how many times you place the order, because if the company never ships it or they ship it to the wrong address, you will never receive it. So, it doesn't matter how many times the TSH places an order with the thyroid gland to produce more hormones; if the thyroid doesn't respond to the TSH by shipping the order (releasing enough hormones), or if the thyroid releases enough hormones but they are shipped to the wrong address (not converted/metabolized properly), then inquiring about the order placed (TSH) will do nothing to get you the package (optimal thyroid hormone metabolism). The TSH fluctuates so much throughout the day that using it alone as a diagnostic tool is extremely inadequate.

The most important thing is that your body receives the package (i.e., adequate levels of the biologically active hormone T3). If you placed an order online but never received it and you wanted to get to the bottom of it, your investigation would not illogically start with the question, "Well, let's see, how many times did I call and place the order?" Who cares how many times you called and placed the order. What matters is figuring out why you didn't receive it. Naturally, you would call the company and speak with the shipping department first to try and find out why you did not receive the package (you might confirm the shipping address or confirm a tracking number from them). However, you would not call the company to ask them how many times you placed the order. It is just as ridiculous to rely on a TSH test to assess someone's thyroid status. In fact, it is harmful to the patient, and sometimes people suffer for more than twenty years because of this nonsense.

TSH Suppression

The TSH test is the bane of hypothyroid patients' existence—and the most misused blood test in the history of thyroid treatment. As mentioned before, the TSH is not a thyroid hormone, it is a pituitary hormone whose *only job* is to wake up the thyroid and tell it to produce T4 and T3 when it senses the body is low in these hormones. This is referred to as a closed-loop feedback process because adequate levels of T4 and T3 in the body will automatically shut down the TSH and "suppress" it. Once a person takes thyroid hormone replacement containing T3, the pituitary senses the body has enough thyroid hormones and doesn't need a wake-up call. So the pituitary shuts up and lowers, or stops sending signals to the thyroid gland. When a person gets optimized on T4/T3 combination therapy, their TSH value becomes suppressed, which is absolutely normal and usually goes hand in hand with T4/T3 and T3-only thyroid hormone optimization. However, some endocrinologists and doctors will tell you that having a suppressed TSH is dangerous (details on this in the interviews with Dr. Foresman in appendix 1). A suppressed TSH usually looks something like this on a blood test: TSH result: <0.01 (0.450–4.500).

I have heard all sorts of unfounded reasons for this fear of TSH suppression from doctors, including an endocrinologist who told me, "TSH suppression can cause heart problems and cancer." Yet every hypothyroid person I know who is optimized on a T3-containing prescription and lives a symptom-free life (including myself) has a suppressed TSH. Why is that a common theme? When a hypothyroid patient starts taking thyroid hormones containing T3, the mechanism by which your thyroid is signaled to produce thyroid hormones, TSH, stops sending out the signal; it senses that the body is getting enough thyroid hormones.

In a hypothyroid state, the thyroid is producing inadequate levels of thyroid hormones to satisfy the body's needs. The TSH is constantly trying to tell the thyroid to produce more thyroid hormones when it senses that the body is very low. When the thyroid does not listen to the TSH signal for whatever reasons, the TSH signal can get louder and louder. The TSH is essentially "screaming" at the thyroid gland to do its job. A very high TSH result can be an indicator of hypothyroidism (whether it's sparked by inadequate hormone replacement, Reverse T3, or faulty thyroid gland function).

Let's look at it another way. If you are hypothyroid and need to be on thyroid hormones, your already sluggish, slow thyroid gland has proven it is unable to properly receive and carry out the TSH wake-up call. So, it's futile for the TSH to keep attempting to wake up a comatose thyroid, especially after a person "overrides the TSH" by taking thyroid hormones containing T3. Often, in undertreated hypothyroid people, there will be a low Free T4 and a low Free T3 along with a higher TSH, which, in a lot of cases, basically means the body is begging for thyroid hormones in order to survive.

My TSH has been suppressed for years. TSH suppression is *never a goal*, but it often coincides with thyroid hormone optimization for people who take NDT, T3-only, or a synthetic T4/T3 combo.

> *TSH suppression is never a goal, but it often coincides with thyroid hormone optimization for people on T4/T3 combination treatment (including NDT) and for people on T3-only.*

Following are my hypothyroid blood results from when I was first diagnosed with hypothyroidism. At this point in time, I had never felt worse in my life. You don't have to be a doctor to see how terrible these labs are, and the corresponding levels of T3 you see here are directly related to the onslaught of symptoms I experienced. Even though the two blood draws were taken at different labs with slightly different reference ranges, you can see how drastically low my Free T3 was in both cases. I was severely hypothyroid and had not yet started thyroid hormone replacement.

ELLE—NOVEMBER 2005

(Severely Hypothyroid—not on thyroid hormones)

TEST	RESULT	RANGE	NOTES
Free T3	1.52	(1.80 - 4.20)	below the range
Free T4	1.28	(0.80 - 1.90)	
TSH	1.08	(0.40 - 4.00)	

ELLE—JANUARY 2006

(Severely Hypothyroid—not on thyroid hormones)

TEST	RESULT	RANGE	NOTES
Free T3	2.86	(2.30 - 4.20)	low in the range
Free T4	.075	(0.80 - 2.30)	below the range
TSH	1.56	(0.50 - 5.50)	

Before I was properly tested, doctors solely tested my TSH and told me that I was fine, because my TSH was *within range*. If you look at my TSH results above, the results are definitely within range, but previous doctors were not testing my Free T4 and Free T3 along with the TSH–until I was finally tested properly in November 2005. My body was falling apart rapidly and these *TSH test–reliant doctors* kept sending me away, saying, "Your thyroid is fine, you just need to exercise more and eat less." If just one of those doctors had known about testing Free T3 and how to evaluate it, I wouldn't have gone undiagnosed for as long as I did, nor suffered for as long as I did.

Why Test Free T4?

If Free T3 is really the ultimate marker of how well someone is doing and feeling, then why test Free T4?

- A very high T4 on a blood test when someone is on thyroid hormone replacement—or the natural over-production of T4 in someone who is not taking thyroid hormones—can indicate an *overactive* thyroid, hyperthyroidism.
- A high Free T4 on a blood test of someone on NDT could partially indicate a Reverse T3 problem (T4 to T3 conversion issue).

Below are the exact same blood tests as my hypothyroid blood panel, except the below tests were taken a few years later, when I was *fully optimized on NDT* and feeling wonderful—every hypothyroid symptom gone! At the time of the tests below I was on 3-3.5 grains of NDT.

ELLE—MAY 2009 *(Optimized on 3–3.5 grains of NDT)*

TEST	RESULT	RANGE	NOTES
Free T3	372	(230–420)	over mid-range
Free T4	1.4	(0.8–1.8)	mid-range
TSH	<0.01		"suppressed"

ELLE—SEPTEMBER 2010 *(Optimized on 3–3.5 grains of NDT)*

TEST	RESULT	RANGE	NOTES
Free T3	370	(230–420)	over mid-range
Free T4	1.4	(0.8–1.8)	mid-range
TSH	<0.03		"suppressed"

You will notice that in both cases my TSH is "suppressed," meaning the pituitary TSH signal was shut down—no more "wake-up calls" being sent to my thyroid gland. My pituitary continually sensed that there was enough T4 and T3 in my blood so it stopped trying to signal my thyroid to produce more thyroid hormones.

Reverse T3—Your Body's Emergency Alarm

Earlier I mentioned that the *remaining percentage of T4 not converted into T3, converts into something called Reverse T3 (RT3)*, a normal process by which the extra T4 in the body is cleared out. Levels of RT3 fluctuate throughout the day and are considered normal, except when too much RT3 is produced. RT3 is similar to T3, except RT3 is *biologically inactive*. Producing too much RT3 will have negative effects on metabolic processes and make someone hypothyroid (whether or not they take thyroid hormones).

Below are my blood results when I discovered I had a Reverse T3 problem. Calculating a ratio between the Free T3 and Reverse T3 yields accurate results in assessing an RT3 problem. A result of 20 or higher is considered healthy. (You can find links to free RT3/Free T3 ratio calculators and instructions on how to calculate the ratio yourself online.)

ELLE—JULY 2011 *(Reverse T3)*

TEST	RESULT	RANGE	NOTES
FREE T3	4.2	(2.3–4.2)	high (normal for some people)
FREE T4	1.7	(0.8–1.8)	high and a red flag
TSH	0.01		"suppressed" (normal for me)
RT3 Ratio: 12.7 not healthy			

Free T3/Reverse T3 Ratio: 20 or higher is considered healthy.
Total T3/Reverse T3 Ratio: 10 and higher is considered healthy.

At the time of this blood draw, I was severely hypothyroid and feeling miserable even though I was on seemingly adequate amounts of thyroid hormone replacement that had worked for about seven years prior to this test. As you can see, the RT3 value above is only a point over the range, but the ratio of 12.7 was a clear indication (along with symptoms,) that I was facing a Reverse T3 problem. Some people have Reverse T3 values "within range" but the ratio between their Free T3 and Reverse T3 implies an RT3 problem, which why it is critical to *evaluate the ratio* between Free T3 and RT3 at the same time and not just rely on the RT3 value on its own.

My Free T4 was 1.7, which is over the mid-range and at the top of the entire range (mid-range is 1.4). This should have been an indication to my doctor that there was some kind of problem. My Free T3 was at the top of the range, which was not unusual for me at the time; however, my Free T4 was over 1.4 and at the top of the range, *which was unusual for me.* That significant change in values should have been a red flag to my doctor to investigate Reverse T3—if only she had known what RT3 was. At the very least, I could've been helped if she had been willing to learn about RT3 and how to treat it, but she wasn't. (More on what to do about RT3 in chapter 4.)

Testing for Hashimoto's Disease (Antibodies TPOAb and TgAb)

Hashimoto's disease is actually *not* a thyroid disease; it is an *autoimmune disease that affects the thyroid.* It is a very common thyroid disorder whereby the immune system attacks the thyroid gland (via antibodies) as if it were a foreign intruder. The immune system will continually attempt to destroy the thyroid gland, and these "attacks" will eventually cause inflammation and the gradual demise of the thyroid gland.

Due to the immune attacks on the thyroid gland, one of the unique characteristics of Hashimoto's is that one day you could feel *hyper*thyroid and a few days later you could feel *hypo*thyroid. Because the attacks cause inflammation of the thyroid gland, discomfort in the neck area is a common symptom, or lumps and nodules can appear on the thyroid gland itself.

HASHIMOTO'S DIAGNOSIS: TWO ANTIBODY TESTS

TPOAb

- This antibody attacks a thyroid enzyme called thyroid peroxidase.
- Usually looks like this on a blood test: range 0–34.
- A result within range indicates an autoimmune response but sometimes can be considered "catching it early before it gets worse." (Thyroid hormone replacement can be avoided and antibody levels can be reduced by adopting a paleo lifestyle!)
- A result over the range and/or very high indicates the patient is likely experiencing full-blown Hashimoto's symptoms. Antibody levels can get as high as 1000+.

TgAb

- This antibody attacks a protein in the thyroid called thyroglobulin, which is crucial to the thyroid-producing T4 and T3 hormones.
- Usually looks like this on a blood test: range 0.0–0.9.
- Let's say the result was <1.0 (less than 1.0). That would mean the patient does not have these antibodies present.

Both of these antibody tests are necessary in diagnosing Hashimoto's, because some people show positive for one and not the other–or both. Since people with untreated Hashimoto's can fluctuate between being hyperthyroid and hypothyroid, using a TSH test would also be useless and misleading. In a Hashimoto's patient, the TSH results can be very high one day, and very low the next. One day, the TSH is screaming at the thyroid to wake up and start working because the pituitary senses a lack of thyroid hormones in the body, and a few days later the TSH is low because the pituitary senses an overproduction of thyroid hormones.

Even after a Hashimoto's patient becomes optimized on thyroid hormone replacement, they can still have high levels of antibodies, which need to be addressed. The presence of thyroid antibodies *is a problem* because they equal inflammation, and inflammation is at the root of many diseases. Grains are a known trigger for Hashimoto's (more on the grains-Hashimoto's connection and treating autoimmunity with a paleo approach in my discussion with Dr. Foresman in appendix 1).

COMMON MISDIAGNOSES WITH HASHIMOTO'S

Because of thyroid fluctuations that people experience with undiagnosed Hashimoto's, sufferers are all too often misdiagnosed with depression, bipolar disorder, or another psychiatric label. Parents of teenage children with undiagnosed Hashimoto's might excuse their teenagers' erratic behavior as "classic teenage puberty drama." Everyone who walks into a doctor's office complaining of depression or any other emotional/psychiatric issues should immediately have their thyroid levels tested, including the two Hashimoto's antibody tests.

"It is not uncommon for women with thyroid problems to suffer from depression. One explanation for this is that the most biologically active form of thyroid hormone, T3, is actually a bona fide neurotransmitter that regulates the action of serotonin, norepinephrine, and GABA (gamma aminobutyric acid), an inhibitory neurotransmitter that is important for quelling anxiety."

—Christiane Northrup, MD, drnorthrup.com

The Suffering Can Stop

There's no denying that the symptoms of thyroid disease are brutal, and it can be hard to get a helpful doctor. But the good news is that the suffering you're going through can stop much sooner than you imagine. Just a couple of weeks on the right medication can get you moving down the path of feeling better. So let's talk medication!

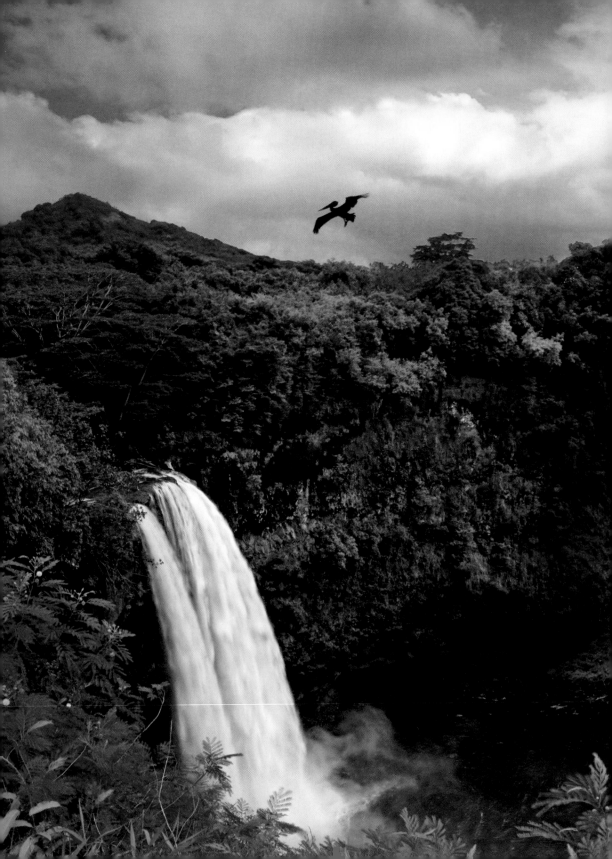

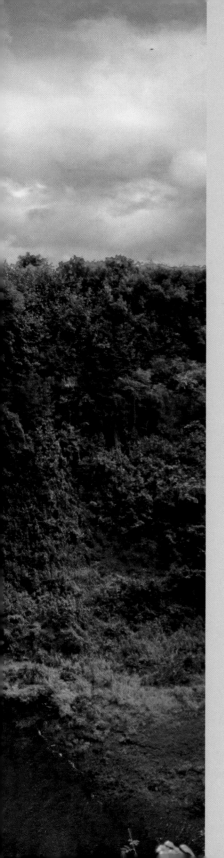

CHAPTER THREE

Fixing Thyroid Issues: Medications and Supplements

*The Paleo Thyroid Solution is a
whole-life approach to health,
but you need to get your nutrient levels
(and sometimes medication) aligned
in order to be successful.
I've been working with supplements
and my own medication for over
a decade now. I am confident that you
and your doctor can find the right
dosages that will make you feel vibrant
and healthy and like yourself again.*

Thyroid Hormone Replacement Options

- Synthetic T4 (levothyroxine)
- Natural Desiccated Thyroid (NDT) is a T4/T3 combination made from desiccated pig thyroid glands. Each "grain" (or 60–65 mg pill) of NDT has about 38 mcg of T4 and 9 mcg of T3. It is the only thyroid hormone replacement option that contains T1, T2, and calcitonin. (There is no evidence suggesting that the presence of these three components are necessary for longevity, overall health, or thyroid hormone health and metabolism.)
- Synthetic T4/T3 combination (levothyroxine/liothyronine sodium), and each hormone value can be adjusted by the doctor to suit the individual needs.
- Synthetic T3 (liothyronine sodium) comes in regular form (direct) or sustained-release (SRT3).

COMMON *STARTING* DOSES FOR THYROID HORMONE REPLACEMENT

- T4-only: 50 mcg if patient is young, 25 mcg if patient is older (above fifty)
- NDT: 1/2 grain (30 mg) to 1 grain (60–65 mg)
- Synthetic T4/T3: Doctor can adjust both values for the patient's individual needs
- T3-only: 5–25 mcg

Most Popular Brand of T4
> **Synthroid**

Most Popular Brand of T3
> **Cytomel**

Most Popular Brands of NDT
> **NP Thyroid** (Acella Pharmaceuticals)
> A generic brand of desiccated thyroid. You can take the pills sublingually, which is an option patients like; I preferred it when I took NDT.

Nature-Throid (RLC Labs)

Patients might want to chew up the tablets before swallowing them, as it may assist in breaking down the cellulose filler in the pills.

WP Thyroid (RLC Labs)

Considered the option for chemically sensitive patients, RLC Labs claims that WP Thyroid is *gluten-free* and contains NDT (porcine) with only three fillers.

Others NDT brands

Armour Thyroid (USA)

Thyroid-S (Thailand)

Thiroid (Thailand)

Thyroid (Canada)

T4-ONLY TREATMENT (LEVOTHYROXINE)

While T4-only treatment is the easiest to dose (usually once a day, in the morning), it comes with its share of serious problems.

- Doctors who offer T4-only treatment as the first choice for thyroid hormone replacement often do not understand the relevance of testing Free T3; therefore, that patient who is on T4-only treatment might be getting only their TSH and Free T4 tested, which will not accurately assess how that patient is truly doing in terms of thyroid hormone metabolism and T4 to T3 conversion.
- T4-only treatment might work at first, but many people have had T4-only treatment fail and stop working for them.
- Although the thyroid gland dispenses T4 into the bloodstream in more abundant amounts than T3, the thyroid gland is still giving us direct T3. Our own bodies don't completely rely on the conversion from T4 to T3. A combination of T4 and T3 is the choice that best mimics the natural endocrine process.
- Sometimes T4-only treatment never works for a patient until they add T3 to their T4 dose or switch over to NDT.

NDT TREATMENT (NATURAL DESICCATED THYROID)

NDT treatment is an excellent choice for hypothyroid patients, and has been since the late 1800s when it was discovered. It is considered the most natural thyroid hormone replacement option available. Even though NDT treatment works well for a lot of people, there are variables involved with each patient. Some patients might need to add extra T4 or extra T3 to their NDT treatment in order to get optimized on the correct levels of hormones. There are some people who are very sensitive, or sometimes allergic, to the fillers used in NDT pills, in which case a compounded synthetic T4/T3 combo might be more optimal. NDT is produced from slaughtered pigs; people who have ethical issues with killing animals or religious reasons to not consume pork might not choose NDT.

A Brief History of NDT and T4

In 1891 an English physician pioneered the treatment of endocrine disorders by injecting hypothyroid patients with sheep thyroid extract—and it worked! Later on, pigs became the main source of thyroid hormone replacement, and one of the most optimal thyroid hormone replacement options today is the use of desiccated pig thyroid gland, referred to as NDT. Until the 1950s, NDT, which contains T4 and T3, was the standard hormone replacement option for hypothyroidism.

*In 1914 a man who later discovered the activity of cortisone first isolated the thyroid hormone T4. Around 1926 synthetic T4 was produced and used in an experiment with two women whose hypothyroid symptoms improved with the administration of T4. In the 1950s pharmaceutical companies could not patent NDT, **but they could patent T4**, so they did, igniting one of the most profitable marketing campaigns to date. According to IMS Health, the top pill popped in America is Synthetic T4, with 23 million brand-name (Synthroid) prescriptions alone filled every year.*

*The campaign **selling point** was that Synthroid (T4-only) was the only recommended treatment for hypothyroidism and that NDT was unstable and uncontrollable. Hypothyroid patients began to suffer at the hands of this* *unethical business move for the sake of profit ever since Synthroid was created in 1958. Patients are still suffering under the outdated and false premise from a pharmaceutical company that continues to infect the practices taught in medical school.*

While Synthroid was being promoted as the one-size-fits-all medication for hypothyroidism, false and negative claims about NDT emerged in several medical articles and journals. They were later identified as hoaxes, but the damage was done; NDT became an exile until its resurgence in the 1990s. In fact, even today most endocrinologists will still tell you that NDT is unstable and meant for pigs not humans, and they do not prescribe it to their thyroid patients. I challenge any reader to pick up the phone and call five random endocrinologists in any United States city and ask the nurse if the doctor prescribes NDT for treating hypothyroidism. It's almost a guarantee that they will say no.

T3-ONLY TREATMENT

T3-only treatment can be considered the last order of business when it comes to thyroid hormone replacement therapy. This treatment is reserved for people who have problems converting T4 to T3 (or some other underlying issues like Lyme disease or other chronic infection that can inhibit T4 to T3 conversion). Sometimes the underlying factors that can cause a conversion problem can be corrected, and then the patient can go back on a T4/T3 combination.

NDT Dosing Protocols

The typical starting dose for desiccated thyroid is one grain (60–65 mg). A lot of people find it beneficial to increase every two weeks in 1/2-grain increments, because the feedback loop of suppression that starts when you commence thyroid hormone replacement can cause further hypothyroid symptoms. One of the biggest mistakes doctors and patients make is that they wait too long in between increases, and sometimes patients experience more hypothyroid symptoms because they are on *too low a dose for too long*. Once a patient reaches the 2 grain mark, it is wise to increase by 1/4 grain increments, until the optimal dose is reached. This conservative approach gives the T4 enough time to build up and offers you and your doctor an accurate picture of the T4 conversion results (which sometimes can take three to six weeks). This process is very individual and can be assessed by the elimination of hypothyroid symptoms affecting body temperature, blood pressure, and pulse, along with checking labs to compare how you are feeling with the corresponding blood results and Free T3 levels. With NDT sometimes just a 1/4 grain increase can make the difference between remaining hypothyroid and being optimized at the right dose. So, any doctor who says, "Your T3 must be at value *x*" is uninformed and does not understand that the elimination of symptoms is more important than trying to target a specific lab result. (You should *run* from such a doctor.) When using compounded T4/T3, sometimes just a 1–2 microgram adjustment can be the determining factor in optimization for a patient. *Dosing and lab values are individual—period.*

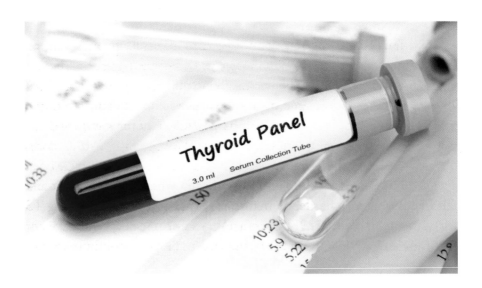

THE PALEO THYROID SOLUTION

Sublingual vs. Swallowing NDT or T3-Only

Some brands of NDT can be taken sublingually (i.e., they dissolve under the tongue). I have always taken my thyroid hormone replacement sublingually; I did it when I was on NDT, and I continue to do it on T3-only. Upon taking NDT or T3-only sublingually, the saliva will start the digestive process by breaking down larger molecules into smaller molecules thereby assisting the absorption into your bloodstream via all of the tiny capillaries that line the inside of the mouth. The best way to think about it is that you get more bang for your buck by taking thyroid hormones sublingually, because that not only bypasses the gastric action in your stomach, which could lead to losing some of the ingredients, but it also bypasses the metabolizing action of the liver.

People who I know that are on thyroid hormones and cannot take them sublingually (such as T4-only, synthetic T4/T3 combo, compounded T4/T3, or sustained-release T3-only) can still achieve optimal results. However, if you do swallow your thyroid hormone replacement, then you need to avoid taking estrogen, calcium, or iron at the same time, because they can bind to the thyroid hormones and cancel them out, so to speak.

Most patients are instructed to take their thyroid hormones on an empty stomach and wait an hour afterwards before eating. Some people have found this not to be the case, and they feel taking their NDT with food slows the release of T3 into their bloodstream, offering a more even release throughout the day. While I never swallowed my NDT when I was on it, I noticed that swallowing my T3-only doses did not have the same benefits as taking it sublingually. In fact, I felt a significant decrease in the effects of the T3 when I swallowed it and felt like dosing was harder to manage and gauge when swallowing T3 versus taking it sublingually. There are people on T3-only who have not noticed the same negative effects, but because I did, I continue to take my T3 doses sublingually.

How Many Times a Day Do I Take My Thyroid Medication?

T4-ONLY

T4-only is usually dosed once a day, and the T4, along with the body's needs, will determine when to convert it to T3 throughout the day.

T4/T3 COMBO AND NDT

It is more beneficial to dose T4/T3 combo or NDT more than once a day. T3 peaks within a couple of hours after taking it, and it doesn't last very long. T4 has a much longer "life." Multi-dosing is more in alignment with how the thyroid works naturally. The thyroid gland dispenses direct T3 into our systems, but the thyroid *does not dispense all of the thyroid hormones needed for the entire day in one single blast in the morning*. Furthermore, sometimes the direct T3 in NDT can be too much for the body in one single dose and can induce stress on the adrenal glands. Failing to multi-dose can leave a patient sleepy in the afternoon.

A two to one ratio works well when multi-dosing T4/T3 combo and NDT. For example, if a person is on 3 grains per day, a dosing strategy could be 2 grains in the morning and 1 grain around 3:30 p.m./4:00 p.m. There are other people who do well on split even-dose scenarios (1.5 grains in the morning and 1.5 grains in the afternoon). There are some patients who multi-dose NDT three times a day.

In my opinion, it might make a little more sense to take a larger dose in the morning to prepare the body for a day's worth of activity, and also because cortisol output is reliant on adequate levels of T3 in the blood. (Our largest surge of cortisol happens in the few hours preceding our rise from sleep.) Since direct T3 peaks within a few hours of ingesting it, multi-dosing prevents big spikes of T3 in the system. Again, this process is not only individual but it can always be altered and adjusted as time goes on.

T3-ONLY (DIRECT T3)

In the case of people on T3-only (like myself), dosing three to five times a day is common. T3 spikes within two hours and reaches tissue saturation within four hours, so dosing three to five times a day is most optimal. I currently dose my T3 four times a day.

Many people ask me why a T3-only patient wouldn't just choose the sustained-release version of T3 in favor of direct T3, since it has an easier dosing schedule (usually twice a day). I have communicated with a multitude of patients on T3-only who say the sustained version didn't work well: sustained-release was more difficult to dose, inconsistent, and they felt their bodies needed a quick replacement dose of T3. Many of those people went back on direct T3 and felt better again. I not only prefer to dose sublingually (which you can't do with sustained-release T3), but I also have a sense of overall control with direct T3 *because of its rapid release*. I don't have to worry about mismanaged T3 levels in my body by trusting the sustained-release component to act synergistically with my fluctuating T3 needs. The direct-release T3 allows me to be aware of *how much* I need and *exactly when* I need it, *at all times*.

T3 is extremely reliable and consistent when used conservatively and wisely. I am able to track the ebbs and flows of when T3 rises, maintains, and then dissipates in my body and brain. Direct T3 enables me to notice subtle nuances and adjust my dosages accordingly. I don't trust the sustained-release form to figure all of that out for me; I am an individual with *individual needs*. Sustained-release T3 is designed to release a steady stream of T3 into your system over a certain period of time (six to eight hours). That wouldn't work for me because I have learned that my body doesn't require evenly dosed levels of T3, and as a result I use a tailored-dose strategy. *I need T3 when I need T3*, and those needs vary.

Compare the idea of sustained-release T3 with T4-only. T4 and the body are meant to coincide and convert the T4 into T3 *whenever that particular human needs it*. Sustained-release T3 seems like a one-size-fits-all way of dosing T3, and I cannot imagine it being as dependable as tailoring direct T3 doses to my specific needs.

SUSTAINED-RELEASE T3

Usually taken twice a day and designed to release one dose of sustained-release T3 steadily over six to eight hours.

Do Not Take Your T4/T3 Combo, NDT, or T3-Only Dose the Morning of a Blood Test!

Ingesting any T3-containing hormone replacement before a blood test can throw it off and lead to inaccurate or false results, because the T3 component can spike/peak in your system just a few hours after taking it. And that false "higher Free T3 result" can keep patients undertreated by doctors. The reason we test Free T3 is to see what is unbound and available in the blood, not what we just sent coursing through our veins by ingesting T3 thyroid hormones an hour before a morning blood test. *Free T3 results are most in line with how the patient is feeling.* In order to accurately assess how your symptoms or lack of symptoms relate to thyroid hormone blood results, it's important to write yourself a reminder to not take your morning dose. You can bring it with you to the lab and pop it in your mouth after the blood draw.

Doctors who suggest you take a thyroid dose containing T3 prior to a blood test do not understand the nuances of thyroid hormone replacement optimization.

COMMON THEMES IN PATIENTS OPTIMIZED ON NDT

- TSH is usually suppressed (often a value of 0.01 in a range of 0.450–4.500).
- Free T4 will be mid-range (usually a value of 1.4 in a range of 0.82–1.77).
- Free T3 will be in the top half of the range, often toward the upper end of the range (3.5–4.4 in a reference range of 2.0–4.4).

COMMON THEMES IN PATIENTS OPTIMIZED ON T3-ONLY (DIRECT T3, NOT SLOW-RELEASE T3)

- TSH will be more suppressed than on NDT (a value of 0.006 in a range of 0.450–4.500).
- Free T4 will be suppressed (a value of 0.11 in a range of 0.82–1.77).
- Free T3 is usually *over the top of the range* to compensate for the fact that T3-only patients have no T4 converting into T3. There

are T3-only patients with a Free T3 substantially over the range who are not hyperthyroid or overstimulated in any way.

- Tracking vitals and temperatures is an accurate tool in finding one's optimal T3 dose versus relying on lab result numbers and ranges. I might feel and exhibit hyperthyroid symptoms with a Free T3 at 5.6, but a fellow T3-only patient might feel hypothyroid if their Free T3 drops below 5.6. *Thyroid dosing is an individual process and needs to be treated as such by doctors.*

How Do I Know I Am Optimized on Thyroid Hormone Replacement?

Symptom elimination is truly the ultimate in knowing whether or not you have successfully treated your hypothyroidism. Aside from looking at the common themes I just mentioned, one should be seeking the complete removal of every hypothyroid symptom along with a morning basal body temperature between 97.8°F and 98.2°F, an afternoon temperature of 98.6°F, and healthy blood pressure and heart rate. Sustained energy throughout the day usually corresponds with successful optimization.

It is a very common experience among hypothyroid sufferers that as they get better and better and their symptoms continue to subside, they often realize they had symptoms they were not even aware of. Because hypothyroid patients are often undiagnosed and undertreated for long periods of time, it is a common experience to grow accustomed to feeling terrible, and truly forgetting what it was like to be happy, normal, and thriving. Sometimes hypothyroid patients never felt normal to begin with, so they don't have a proper gauge of what it feels like to be in optimal health until they actually reach it and can then look back with the realization they had actually been suffering for a long time. I know people who lived a crummy existence for eight or twenty years before being diagnosed and/or treated properly.

As a patient starts to feel better along their journey of thyroid hormone replacement they can mistakenly believe they are optimized. It is advantageous to experiment, with your doctor, with dosing and become aware of symptoms and signs along the way so that you can find your perfect dose. Tracking temperatures and vitals during this process is extremely beneficial to reaching optimization.

The way to truly know whether or not you are optimized on thyroid hormone replacement is that when you are optimized, you feel like a million bucks! Check out these "symptoms" of optimization:

- Sustained energy throughout the day
- Mental focus to concentrate for long periods of time
- Simple everyday tasks are no longer overwhelming
- Wonderful, deep sleep and feeling rested and energized upon waking in the morning
- Invigorated by exercise instead of feeling sleepy or exhausted during and/or afterwards
- A sense of purpose again and feeling excited about your future
- A positive outlook and happiness (whereas before those emotions seemed unattainable)
- A healthy sex drive
- Improved memory
- Better muscle recovery after exercise, significant reduction in muscle stiffness/soreness
- Healthy, vibrant skin and hair
- Normal menstrual periods and overall gynecological health

How Do I Find a Doctor Who Is Truly Informed?

Over the course of ten-plus years, I found it extremely difficult to find doctors who were well trained when it comes to thyroid hormone replacement and optimization. Usually the doctors who understand all of the nuances are those who have gone above and beyond the standard MD license by seeking further medical training after medical school, and these doctors actually spend more time with patients (integrative physicians, functional medicine doctors, Doctors of Osteopathy, and anti-aging doctors).

In choosing a doctor, the most important criteria are through assessing the following variables. You can always call any doctor's office and ask the nurse to get back to you on these questions.

- Does the doctor routinely test Free T3 or just test TSH and Free T4?
- For thyroid patients does the doctor prescribe and have patients currently on NDT or just T4-only/Synthroid?
- Does the doctor treat patients by the elimination of symptoms along with bloodwork or rely on blood results alone?
- Does the doctor test for and understand how to treat Reverse T3, and if so, what is the usual protocol for fixing it? Has the doctor ever had a patient successfully recover from a Reverse T3 problem?
- Does the doctor prescribe T3-only to patients if required?

Even though I have called doctors' offices and received the "correct responses," you still might meet a doctor in person only to have them rely on labs alone without listening to you or factoring in your symptoms at all. And they might be clueless as to how to prescribe and manage NDT and/or T3-only. It happens. Only until you speak with a doctor face-to-face or over the phone will you know how they treat thyroid patients. If you are unsure or skeptical about a doctor's approach to treating your thyroid problem, move on and keep looking.

The NTH (Natural Thyroid Hormones) Yahoo group (a patient-to-patient forum which anyone can join on Yahoo.com), has compiled a "Good Doctor List" submitted by patients since 2006. It includes doctor descriptions (bad and good) of doctors in each state.

- -

Patient (and Doctor) Mistakes

- *Staying on a **starting dose** for too long, which can make someone feel even more hypothyroid than when they first started thyroid hormones.*
- *Believing hyperthyroid symptoms are from too much thyroid medication, when the symptoms could be stemming from insufficient adrenals and/or low iron.*

It is *extremely rare* to find a doctor who understands how to correct a Reverse T3 problem and who understands the nuances of T3-only dosing (especially direct T3). Most doctors only add direct T3 to a T4 prescription, and rarely do MDs prescribe T3-only. Unfortunately, this has led to many patients taking their health into their own hands and dosing and doctoring themselves, as I did. I wish more doctors would take heed of Pfizer's own medical literature on Cytomel (T3) to help patients who have Reverse T3 problems and want to use T3-only to fix it. Pfizer states in their own literature on Cytomel that T3 can be used when a patient either cannot convert T4 to T3 or does not respond positively to T4 or T4/T3 combination therapy. Some patients cannot resolve RT3 by just lowering their T4 and increasing their T3. Some patients can only resolve it by going on T3-only for eight to twelve plus weeks. Some people remain on T3-only after the RT3 problem is corrected (as I did), and some have gone back on NDT or a T4/T3 combo successfully (which I will eventually attempt myself).

Key Vitamin/Mineral/Hormone Factors Related to Thyroid Function

SELENIUM

Required for the conversion of T4 into T3. A selenium deficiency can manifest with hypothyroid symptoms.

Deficiency Symptoms

- Heavy whitening of the fingernail beds
- Low immunity (more colds and flus)
- Constant fatigue
- Brain fog
- Reproductive issues
- Hypothyroidism
- Reverse T3 problem (inability to convert T4 to T3)

Why Might Deficiency Occur?

- Lack of selenium in the soil. Selenium must be present in the soil to show up in our food. It isn't created out of thin air.
- Insufficient intake of selenium-rich foods.
- Intestinal disorders, like Crohn's disease, ulcerative colitis, and celiac, reduce the absorption of selenium from foods.
- Consuming grains on a regular basis can also inhibit the absorption of nutrients like selenium.

Where to Get Selenium

Brazil nuts (one or two a day are enough to improve selenium status), wild salmon, kidneys, cremini and shiitake mushrooms, lamb, turkey, shrimp, cod, halibut, and egg yolks are all good sources of selenium.

Supplements: Selenomethionine is the form found in plants. Selenocysteine is found in animals.

Testing

Many years ago I discovered that I had a selenium deficiency, which could have caused my hypothyroidism in the first place and/or was a main culprit behind my Reverse T3 problem. I took a popular micronutrient test by SpectraCell Laboratories that measures how micronutrients are actually functioning within the white blood cells. Results help with nutritional assessment for a wide variety of clinical conditions, general wellness, and the prevention of chronic diseases. Aside from a selenium deficiency, my results showed that I also had a deficiency in coenzyme Q10 and B12.

Dosage

A safe supplemental dose appears to be 200–400 mcg per day, but there's very little evidence of selenium toxicity from a diet high in selenium-rich foods. So that Brazil nut–encrusted salmon kidney in shiitake/cremini mushroom sauce with a turkey egg omelet should be worry-free.

MAGNESIUM

Everyone touts its importance; yet, few seem to get enough through diet, and many hypothyroid patients are lacking in this mineral. Low intakes are being linked to type 2 diabetes, metabolic syndrome, osteoporosis, heart disease, asthma, and colon cancer.

Deficiency Symptoms (Just Some of Them)

- Insulin resistance
- Constipation
- Migraines
- Restless leg syndrome
- Muscle cramping
- Heart palpitations
- Hypertension
- Fibromyalgia

Why Might Deficiency Occur?

- Lack of magnesium in the soil.
- Lack of magnesium-rich foods in the diet, particularly plant foods. Animal foods are relatively magnesium-poor, but plants

tend to be magnesium-rich. How many people do you know who really eat *lots* of leafy greens?

- Removal of magnesium from drinking water. I suspect magnesium-rich water (as opposed to purified, depleted modern water) was how our hunter-gatherer ancestors got a lot of their magnesium.
- Too much calcium in the diet.

Where to Get Magnesium

- Leafy greens, especially Swiss chard and spinach.
- Nuts, seeds, dark chocolate, espresso, and halibut.
- Mineral water. One brand of fizzy water, Gerolsteiner, is particularly high in magnesium. Or you could find a spring nearby for some real (free) spring water.
- Supplements: The chelated magnesiums (those ending in "-ate," like citrate, glycinate, or taurate) tend to be the best absorbed.

Testing Magnesium

Magnesium RBC ("Red Blood Cell") should be mid-range or a little higher.

Dosage

The daily minimum dose is 400 mg. You can ingest magnesium in pill form, but there are also a variety of chelated magnesium drinks on the market. My favorite is Natural Calm by Natural Vitality company.

B12 AND HOMOCYSTEINE (AND OTHER B VITAMINS)

Vitamin B12 is important for protein metabolism and assists in the formation of red blood cells. This essential vitamin is critical for solving adrenal fatigue along with several metabolic functions, including enzyme production, DNA synthesis, hormone balance, and maintaining healthy nervous and cardiovascular systems.

Headaches

Lethargy

Infertility

Brain fog

Anxiety and/or depression

Tingling in extremities

Difficulty breathing

Autism spectrum disorder in children

Why Might Deficiency Occur?

Because hypothyroidism negatively affects digestion, often hypothyroid patients have issues absorbing nutrients like B vitamins, B12 in particular. The body needs adequate thyroid hormones to absorb and "hold onto" B12. Consuming grains on a regular basis can also inhibit the absorption of nutrients like B12. Even people who eat plenty of the richest sources of B12 (animals) can have a deficiency.

MTHFR and Homocysteine Connection

Methylenetetrahydrofolate reductase mutation test is used to detect two common mutations in the MTHFR gene that is associated with elevated levels of homocysteine in the blood. Most doctors do not routinely order this test, but it might be appropriate in understanding why a patient has elevated homocysteine levels.

Healthy MTHFR Gene Benefits:
- *MTHFR enzyme works with and breaks down folate vitamins.*
- *Those folate vitamins help convert homocysteine to another amino acid called methionine.*
- *The body uses methionine to make proteins, process fats, maintain and repair cells, along with creating and breaking down brain chemicals.*
- *Methionine helps with inflammation.*

Defective/Mutated MTHFR Gene Downsides:
- *MTHFR enzyme functions perform sluggishly, which can affect the breakdown of toxins or heavy metals.*
- *MTHFR enzyme won't break down folate vitamins properly, which can cause high homocysteine (high homocysteine can increase risk of heart disease and more).*
- *Homocysteine is scantily converted to glutathione (your body's main antioxidant and detoxifier).*

Methylation

Methylation is a vitamin-requiring process in the body that is critical for supporting various aspects of physical and mental health, including normalizing gene expression. Methylation occurs constantly and helps the body to repair DNA regularly. However, when methylation processes slow down, an increase in the breakage of DNA strands occurs. Poor methylation can promote inflammation and poor detoxification in the body.

Where to Get B12
- Liver, sardines, and salmon rank highest, with liver reigning supreme. There are no vegetarian sources.
- Supplements: For B12, methylcobalamin is probably the best. If you are recovering from hypothyroidism and adrenal issues, taking a B-complex supplement one to two times a day can help improve skin quality/tone, repair the adrenals, improve immunity, assist metabolism, and improve emotional health.

Testing B12
Generally aim for the top part of the range. If the range is something like 100–900, then 800 would be optimal, and anything below 400/350 could result in symptoms.

Testing *homocysteine* levels is considered a better way to measure B12 adequacy because homocysteine will go up about a year before B12 levels drop. Elevated homocysteine levels have been linked to increased risk of heart disease and strokes. High levels may also affect blood platelets and increase the risk of clot formation.

Dosage

Among the variety of forms of B12, the one considered most absorbable is called *methylcobalamin* in either liquid sublingual form or sublingual lozenges. (There are also B12 shots available through doctors' offices and some pharmacies.) A good place to start for raising B12 levels is 500 mcg per day. B12 sublingual administration will bypass the intestinal tract and pass directly into the bloodstream.

If you eat animal products regularly and liver occasionally, you'll be getting plenty of B12 in your diet. There is no need to supplement if you have none of the symptoms listed above. But if you have some of the symptoms or you have gastrointestinal issues or hypothyroidism that may be compromising your ability to absorb vitamin B12, consider getting your levels tested.

Other B Vitamins

The vast array of B vitamins helps convert food to fuel. The B vitamins help support our levels of energy, immunity, heart health, emotional well-being, metabolism, and adrenal function.

- Thiamine (B1): Needed for our body to process carbohydrates and sugars.
- Riboflavin (B2): Helps process amino acids and fats. Higher doses have shown to reduce migraines.
- Niacinamide (B3): Helps with energy and essential for DNA repair. Plays a role in gland and liver function. In niacin form it can cause flushing (prickly heat sensation to the face and upper body).
- Pyridoxine (B6): Critical for the production and synthesis of numerous body chemicals, including insulin, hemoglobin, neu-

rotransmitters, enzymes, prostaglandins, histamine, dopamine, and adrenaline.

- Pantothenic Acid: Speeds wound healing. Can help allergies and respiratory disorders, skin disorders, and diabetes. Helps reduce cholesterol levels.
- Folic Acid (B9): Lowers risk of heart disease, stroke, and birth defects. Helps the body produce and maintain new cells and prevent changes to DNA that could lead to cancer.
- Biotin: Beneficial for hair, skin, nails, and blood sugar control.
- Choline: Important for normal brain function and plays a role in methylation.
- Inositol: Helpful for depression and anxiety attacks.
- Para-Aminobenzoic Acid (PABA): Considered helpful in treating skin conditions such as vitiligo and maintaining healthy intestinal flora.

IRON

Iron provides life-affirming oxygen to organ systems through its role in red cell production. Iron is an essential protein component for metabolism (low iron levels often go hand in hand with low B12 results). Without adequate iron, muscles lose their tone and elasticity. Low iron can compromise brain function: oxygen supply in the blood is assisted by iron, and the brain uses approximately 20% of the blood oxygen. Proper flow of blood in the brain stimulates cognitive activity.

Ferritin is "iron storage"; it is important to the amount of iron available in the body. Ferritin acts as a buffer against both iron deficiency and iron overload. It stores iron in a non-toxic way, deposits it in a controlled fashion, and then transports it to areas where it is needed. T4 has a hard time converting to T3 when low levels of ferritin are present.

Deficiency Symptoms (Some symptoms mimic hypothyroid symptoms.)
- Light-headedness/dizziness
- Restless leg syndrome
- Heart palpitations (especially upon laying down)

- Shortness of breath
- Feeling like you cannot take a deep enough breath or get enough air
- Exhausted easily/low energy
- Poor recovery after physical exercise
- Weak limbs
- Brain fog/inability to focus
- Feeling stressed/overwhelmed
- Anxious and easily irritated
- Numbness in hands
- Female orgasm contractions feel "weak" and not as strong as before
- Not enough vaginal moisture when aroused (or different consistency than before)

Why Might Deficiency Occur?

Possible causes of low ferritin include intestinal disease, antacids, excessive blood loss, intestinal bleeding, insufficient red meat or iron-rich foods, regular grain consumption, hypothyroidism (body ineffectively absorbs it and also cannot "hold onto" iron).

Where to Get Iron?

- Food sources include meats, organ meats (like liver), green leafy vegetables, blackstrap molasses, and eggs. Cooking foods in a real cast iron skillet also helps.
- Sometimes food does not work in raising iron effectively, and one must take an iron supplement.

Testing

Because inflammation can throw off a ferritin test and make it appear normal, or even high, getting a comprehensive iron panel will be most effective. Below are optimal levels.
- Ferritin: For both men and women 50–100 (common range is 10–150). Ferritin over 100 can indicate inflammation in the body

or indicate ingesting too much iron. High-quality omega-3 fish oil and krill oil can help reduce high ferritin and inflammation. *(If you are allergic to shellfish as I am, you may need to avoid krill oil.)*

- Total Iron Binding Capacity (TIBC): With healthy levels of iron, this will be low in the range, about one quarter above the bottom number in the range you are using (common range is 250–450). TIBC measures whether a protein called transferrin has the capacity to carry iron in the blood. If your result is high, and in the absence of chronic disease, you might be anemic.
- Serum Iron (amount of circulating iron): Around 110 for women, 130 for men (common range is 35–155).
- % Saturation (serum iron divided by your TIBC): Women usually score around 35% and men 40%–45% (common range is 15%–55%).

Dosage

There are various forms of iron (ferrous sulfate, ferrous bisglycinate, ferrous gluconate, ferrous fumarate, etc.). After having several issues with iron over the years and trying various forms of iron, my favorite form is ferrous bisglycinate chelate, always taken with food (and preferably with vitamin C because it helps with absorption).

This form of iron did not constipate me at all, but if for some reason you feel your bowels are sluggish while taking iron, you can always take 400–800 mg of magnesium nightly. *Heads up: Supplementing with iron will turn your stools black in color, and you might notice a tar-like consistency/appearance. This is normal.*

Iron Supplementation Guidelines

How much iron do I need to take, and for how long?

When my ferritin got down to 10 (in a range of 10–150) and I was riddled with restless legs and many other low iron symptoms, I took 150–200 mg of "elemental iron" spread throughout the day in three doses. The amount of elemental iron contained in iron pills will vary. For example, a 325 mg supplement (of ferrous fumarate or ferrous gluconate) actually contains only 100 mg of "elemental iron" per pill. You can always call the supplement company and ask them about this if it is not mentioned on the label.

It can take anywhere from four to twelve-plus weeks to optimize your ferritin levels, depending on how low they were to begin with. When my ferritin was 10, it took me about three months of taking iron every day to optimize my levels. If levels are not severely suboptimal, sometimes a daily multivitamin with iron can bring up levels in four to six weeks. Once iron is optimized, it might benefit menstruating females to take a multivitamin with iron daily on bleeding days.

Should I avoid anything while taking iron?
Avoid taking calcium with iron, and avoid taking iron with your thyroid hormones (iron can bind with the thyroid hormones, rendering them less potent). Ideally, make sure you take your thyroid hormones and iron two to four hours apart. *Take thyroid hormones an hour before taking iron, or several hours after taking iron.* If you take your thyroid hormones sublingually, there will be significantly less interaction; however, some of the thyroid hormone will still be swallowed when taken sublingually, so it's always better to err on the side of caution and distance thyroid hormone ingestion from iron consumption.

How often do I get my iron levels tested?
Every four weeks is conservative and can help avoid overloading on iron, which can be toxic.

DHEA
DHEA (dehydroepiandrosterone) is a hormone produced by our adrenal glands. It functions as a precursor to hormones such as testosterone, estrogen, and others that regulate fat and mineral metabolism, sexual/reproductive function, and energy levels. DHEA levels naturally decline with age, particularly after thirty, which is why DHEA is sometimes referred to as the "youth hormone" and is considered one of the best biochemical biomarkers of chronological age. Low levels of DHEA can cause hor-

monal imbalance and contribute to adrenal insufficiency/fatigue.

DHEA has demonstrated protective effects for various cancers and is helpful for age-related issues by sharpening memory, enhancing immune function, energy, smooth skin, cardiovascular health, and weight loss, and easing tired muscles.

Deficiency Symptoms

- Fatigue
- Decreased muscle mass and strength
- Low sex drive for men and women (For men, sometimes the absence of an erection upon waking in the morning can be an indicator of low DHEA.)
- Low immunity
- Disrupted sleep
- Aching joints/muscles
- Depression
- Decrease in bone density
- Menopausal symptoms in older women

Why Might Deficiency Occur?

Non–primal/paleo lifestyle and high stress levels contribute to low DHEA levels, because the adrenals can't produce enough DHEA when stressed. Hypothyroid patients are susceptible to low DHEA because of the thyroid-adrenal connection (adrenals overrespond and exhaust DHEA levels due to the lack of thyroid hormones in the body). Chronic stress and/or hypothyroidism = stressed adrenals = low DHEA. Medications such as insulin and corticosteroids can also decrease DHEA. Low DHEA is an indicator that you might not be able to tolerate much exercise.

Supplementing with DHEA

DHEA supplementation strengthens the immune system, builds adrenal glands, provides more energy, improves mood and memory, builds strength and muscle, increases sex drive, boosts anti-aging, helps with depression, helps one maintain a healthy weight. I experienced very low DHEA twice during my bouts of hypothyroidism, and I feel a 180° difference in my overall energy, mood, libido, skin quality, and fat-burning abilities when my DHEA is optimal.

Testing

Upon oral administration, DHEA is mostly converted to DHEA-sulfate, which circulates in the blood far longer than DHEA. Circulating DHEA-sulfate acts as a reserve upon which tissues can draw and is a good way to measure available DHEA in the body.

Because lab reference ranges vary, shooting for a result above mid-range is good. Extremely high DHEA can indicate the adrenals are compensating for a problem or you are supplementing too much. In general, a blood result of 250–450 (depending on the range; common range is 40–325, so aim for a value in the top third of whatever range your lab uses) can be considered optimal for men and women. Lab range example: If the range was 57–279, then mid-range to 250 would be optimal.

Dosage

- Dosing for women: 10–25 mg or more per day
- Dosing for men: 25–50 mg or more per day

VITAMIN D

Even though it's referred to as a vitamin, vitamin D is actually a pro-hormone. The body can produce its own vitamin D through the action of sunlight on the skin, while vitamins are nutrients that are not created by the body and have to be acquired through diet or supplements. Vitamin D regulates the levels of calcium and phosphate in the bloodstream, and it promotes the mineralization and growth of bones, working together with calcium, vitamin A, and vitamin K2. And vitamin D reduces systemic, chronic inflammation.

Vitamin D helps regulate growth in virtually every cell of your body and prevents a variety of diseases. Unfortunately, today's indoor lifestyles result in widespread vitamin D deficiency, which can significantly increase cancer risk by compromising the function of the p53 "spell-checker" gene, which is responsible for regulating healthy cell division. Epidemiology suggests links between vitamin D deficiency and most cancers, including breast, colorectal and most of the major ones. Vitamin D deficiency can also cause cardiovascular illness, cognitive impairment, and renal difficulties.

Vitamin D, crucial to thyroid hormone metabolism, needs to be present in adequate amounts when T3 "punches in" to work (inside the cell). Consider vitamin D the keeper of the "punch card machine," so if vitamin D is not present, T3 cannot affect that cell, or "punch in." Remember, when you don't punch in to work, you don't get paid. If T3 cannot affect the cells properly, you will be hypothyroid.

People with hypothyroidism are often deficient in vitamin D, regardless of sun exposure. Low vitamin D can contribute to low thyroid function. Low levels of vitamin D might make the thyroid more susceptible to irritation from chemicals in the environment, such as fluoride and chlorine. Researchers have discovered a link between vitamin D deficiency and Hashimoto's disease. If vitamin D is not optimal, thyroid hormones might not work well because, as mentioned, vitamin D has to be present in adequate amounts when the T3 "punches in" to work. (The same applies for levels of cortisol and iron.) Vitamin D has the ability to reduce the risk of thyroid cancer.

Deficiency Symptoms

- Hypothyroidism
- Excess weight or obesity
- General malaise or depression
- Achy bones
- Excessive sweating (particularly sweaty head/forehead)
- Weakness (muscular and or/general exhaustion)
- Rickets (in cases of severe vitamin D deficiency)

Why Might Deficiency Occur?

Lack of regular sun exposure is the most common cause. However, people who get regular sun exposure can still be deficient, so it's always important to confirm levels through testing. Hypothyroidism can cause issues with proper absorption in the body and hold onto a variety of nutrients, including vitamin D. Gut issues, such as Crohn's disease, Irritable bowel syndrome (IBS), celiac disease, and leaky gut syndrome, can also inhibit absorption.

Where to Get Vitamin D

Food sources include sardines, wild salmon, caviar, mackerel, herring, catfish, and eggs. Also cod liver oil.

Testing Vitamin D

It's called the 25-hydroxy vitamin D test. A result between 70 and 90 or 100 is considered optimal (common range is 30–100). A result below 50 is considered deficient.

Dosage

For supplementation, you should be looking for vitamin D as D3, or cholecalciferol. To maintain adequate levels, 1,000–2,000 IUs per day. In order to raise inadequate levels, supplementing between 2,000 and 5,000 IUs per day should be sufficient. If there is a severe deficiency, your doctor might suggest 25,000 IUs or more.

IODINE

Iodine is a trace mineral with big implications for our health, especially for the thyroid.

Deficiency Symptoms

- Hypothyroidism
- Goiter (enlarged, visible thyroid gland)
- Cretinism (congenital abnormal neurodevelopment in a child)

Removal of iodized salt from the diet. Most table salt is iodized with the minimum required dose, but when people switch to a whole foods, paleo eating plan, they'll often reduce their salt intake and switch to sea salt (which contains trace minerals but insignificant amounts of iodine).

Lack of iodine in the soil. Although iodine concentration remains pretty constant throughout the ocean, iodine content of soil varies dramatically by region, with some areas having so little that they've earned the term "Goiter Belt." Coastal areas tend to have higher soil iodine levels, due to absorption from atmospheric iodine (which in turn comes from the ocean), but very little solid data exists on the iodine content of soil by region.

Insufficient intake of iodine-rich foods, like seaweed and seafood.

Excessive intake of goitrogen-rich foods (raw cruciferous vegetables), which can interfere with iodine uptake by the thyroid gland.

Where to Get Iodine

- Food sources include basically any creature that lives in the ocean: fish, shellfish, crustaceans. Iodine content of fish varies, but pollock, codfish, and abalone rank highest, but there are lots of other good sources. (Cooking method will also determine iodine content, with boiling losing the most and frying retaining the most. Grilling retains far more iodine than boiling, and just a little less than frying, so that's probably a nice middle ground between boiling and fish sticks. Iodine in the boiling water, however, accounts for most of the lost iodine, so you could always drink or use the water. Raw seafood will retain the most iodine.) Also seaweed, especially hijiki and kelp (or kombu), and pastured egg yolks.
- Popular supplements include kelp supplements, Lugol's solution, Iodoral, and Iosol.

Testing

Sometimes hypothyroid patients make the mistake of thinking that iodine will solve their hypothyroidism, and they start taking larger doses of iodine without testing for a deficiency. I almost made this mistake but wised up quickly and got tested. It turned out that I did not have an iodine deficiency after all.

Whole body sufficiency for iodine can be assessed by taking an iodine/iodide loading test. The test consists of ingesting iodine tablets (included with the test) and collecting urine in a container for twenty-four hours after ingesting the tablets. The most popular tests are from Hakala and Doctor's Data. For more information on iodine and hypothyroidism, refer to my interview with Dr. Foresman in the appendix on page 253.

Dosage

The Recommended Daily Allowance (RDA) is 150 mcg. Seaweed-eating Japanese populations often get upwards of 12.5 mg (or 12,500 mcg) per day, while the general Japanese population gets between 1 and 2 mg per day. While 150 mcg should be the minimum, if you're feeling any of the deficiency symptoms, consider increasing your intake with food sources. Other than including the RDA minimum of 150 mcg into one's diet through a multivitamin, other supplementation, or food sources, iodine can be harmful in high doses if one does not have a true iodine deficiency. Increased iodine consumption in supplemental form can cause problems for people with Hashimoto's because it can instigate autoimmune attacks on the thyroid gland.

OTHER ESSENTIAL FACTORS

These are nutrients and factors that are either difficult or very expensive to test, but they're still important to include in your diet!

Coenzyme Q-10

Found in every cell of our bodies. Found in large amounts in our heart, liver, kidney and pancreas. Our bodies produce it because we need it for cell growth and maintenance. It is considered an antioxidant and helps enzymes work to digest food and perform other bodily processes. Helps protect the heart and skeletal muscles, boost energy and speeds recovery from exercise. Strengthens the immune system. Supplementation is used in treating congestive heart failure, chest pain, and high blood pressure. CoQ10 can be used for other heart and blood vessel conditions. It is important for thyroid and adrenal health. Hypothyroid patients might be deficient in CoQ10.

Zinc

An important trace mineral essential for our bodies and brains to stay healthy. It is found in cells throughout our bodies. Zinc is essential for the body to grow and develop properly during pregnancy, infancy, and childhood. Zinc is needed for optimal immune function, healing wounds, detoxification, blood clotting, and thyroid function. It is essential to brain health and more. Zinc can boost the immune system, treat the common cold, help acne, and help with vision, night blindness, ear infections, asthma, diabetes, eczema, Alzheimer's disease, tinnitus, ADHD, and eating disorders. Low levels of zinc are linked to hypothyroidism, HIV, depression, type 2 diabetes, sickle cell disease, hair loss, lethargy, impotence/infertility, and impaired conversion of T4 to T3. Thyroid hormones are essential for absorbing zinc. Hair loss, known to go along with hypothyroidism, can be associated with a zinc deficiency. Too much zinc can suppress thyroid function.

Vitamin C (Ascorbic Acid)

A water-soluble vitamin and antioxidant needed for the growth and repair of tissues in our bodies. Builds collagen and maintains connective tissue. Our bodies cannot make vitamin C on their own and we don't store it, so we need to get it from our diet or through supplementation. Fruits and vegetables contain large amounts of this vitamin. Vitamin C helps with the absorption of iron, and it also counters the free radicals caused by iron. It is helpful in reducing adrenal stress and generally supports the adrenal glands—the adrenals use more vitamin C than another part of the body. Vitamin C plays a role in thyroid hormone function, because it reduces stress on the thyroid caused by foreign toxins and other harmful free radicals.

Alpha-Lipoic Acid (ALA)

This antioxidant assists in converting blood sugar into available energy, so people with insulin resistance or diabetes could benefit. Many (and perhaps most) antioxidants are insulin-sensitizing agents. They increase the effects of insulin, one of which is the removal of glucose from the blood, so you need less insulin to remove the same amount of glucose. In other words, the same amount of insulin removes even more glucose. If you're lean, if you're perfectly insulin sensitive, if you're walking around with optimal blood glucose levels, consuming an insulin-sensitizing agent may be too much of a good thing, it could make you hypoglycemic. However, if you are insulin resistant/obese/type 2 diabetic/hypoglycemic, then more insulin sensitivity will improve your health.

Testing for Insulin Resistance and Type 2 Diabetes

How do you know if you are insulin resistant or have type 2 diabetes? Aside from one obvious symptom of not being able to lose weight and burn fat, talk to your doctor about ordering the Hemoglobin A1c test (HbA1c). This test reflects your average blood glucose level for the past two to three months to determine if you are insulin resistant or have type 2 diabetes and might benefit from supplementing ALA.

For people without diabetes, the normal range for the HbA1c test is between 4% and 5.6%. Hemoglobin A1c levels between 5.7% and 6.4% indicate insulin resistance and an increased risk of type 2 diabetes; levels of 6.5% or higher indicate diabetes. While mainstream medicine might suggest that a result of 5.7% is considered normal, Dr. Foresman suggests that an HbA1c result over 5.2% is a major red flag and anyone with a result over 5.2% should take a serious look at their carbohydrate/sugar consumption.

Even though I had fixed my thyroid issue, adopted a paleo/primal lifestyle, lost the majority of the weight I had gained, and reached proper nutrient levels, my HbA1c result was 5.7%, which indicates insulin resistance and a

prediabetic state. I thought I had "stalled" on weight loss for some other rea-
son, until my HbA1c result confirmed insulin resistance. Likely leftover from
the hypothyroid disease state my body had previously been in along with my
former sugar addiction and excess carb consumption, I needed to further, and
significantly, adjust my diet in order to nip insulin resistance in the bud for
good. More of this in paleo/primal chapter 5.

Thyroid Health and Sex Hormones (Men and Women)

Since thyroid hormones are responsible for the production and regulation of sex hormones, hypothyroidism often affects sex hormones negatively, resulting in deficiencies/imbalances that can lead to more health problems. You can have your doctor test sex hormones to see where your levels are, but understand that getting your thyroid hormones optimized can correct and reverse hormone imbalances.

I had very *low* testosterone both while I remained undiagnosed with hypothyroidism and again when I experienced Reverse T3 issues. My testosterone was low twice in ten years, and both times it *naturally* came back to normal after getting optimized on thyroid hormone replacement. My female hormones were also "off" while I was severely hypothyroid, and one of the many doctors I saw prescribed progesterone cream based on those blood results—which made everything worse. Finally, an acupuncturist told me to stop the progesterone cream and start thyroid hormone replacement. All of my hormones got back into balance once I was optimized on thyroid hormones.

Taking sex hormones while hypothyroid—especially if you are non-menopausal woman or a male under the age of fifty—is akin to putting a bandage on a symptom that is actually caused by a correctable root problem, hypothyroidism. Getting one's hormones back in order could take three to six-plus months to achieve after starting thyroid hormones, but in my opinion it is worth waiting to see if normal production and rhythm of sex hormones return on their own. Wacky adrenals and blood sugar imbalances also negatively affect sex hormones, so becoming fat adapted by adopting a paleo/primal lifestyle can help bring the symphony of hormonal interactions back in line.

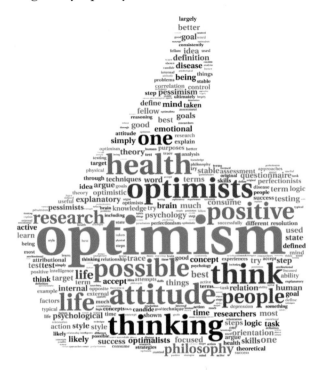

Thyroid Problem-Solving Principles

In order to troubleshoot your thyroid and get it working for you again, you need to follow these problem-solving principles. If you get discouraged or overwhelmed, visit chapter 8 for inspiring stories about people (including me!) who have overcome years of feeling wretched.

DO YOUR OWN RESEARCH

Starting with this book! As you might have already gathered, there are many doctors out there who are uninformed when it comes to thyroid health. It is imperative that you not only become knowledgeable about what is happening to your body, but that you research as much as you can about every aspect of solving the problem, no matter what it is. Had

I allowed doctors to completely control my health, I would probably still be sick today—or maybe even dead. Even if you have a wonderful doctor who has proven to be a great ally in your quest for health in the past, you are still the only one living in your body, and in order to take control of what's happening to it, it is critical that you learn everything you can. If you can read and have internet access (available at most public libraries for free) then you have the ability to research and get to the bottom of any health problem you are experiencing.

There are millions of people already on thyroid hormone replacement who are not feeling great, and many just assume that's the way life is supposed to be, because their doctors keep telling them that their thyroid health is fine! Are you really going to fully trust someone else with your health and potentially spend five to ten or more years with low energy, compromised brain function, and low-grade depression before you are willing to stand up and do something to find the answers? I wouldn't; and I didn't.

There are too many people in our country with diseases and health problems who have no idea what is actually happening in their bodies because they blindly trust that their doctors know what to do. I cannot even count the number of people I have spoken to who are on thyroid hormone replacement, but are completely undertreated, with a myriad of hypothyroid symptoms. Yet, they lack the desire to try to get to the bottom of why they are not feeling well. Take control of your health and body by learning everything you can about thyroid health.

FOLLOW YOUR GUT

Certainly, there are mixed messages out there in the ether when it comes to health problems and the best ways to solve them. I didn't take every piece of advice that I received from fellow hypothyroid patients or online research, but when I did I used my gut and intuition to decipher those suggestions in light of my research. There might be a variety of "correct" ways to go about solving a problem, but I think extensive research, advice from fellow patients and doctors, along with using intuition is a winning combination.

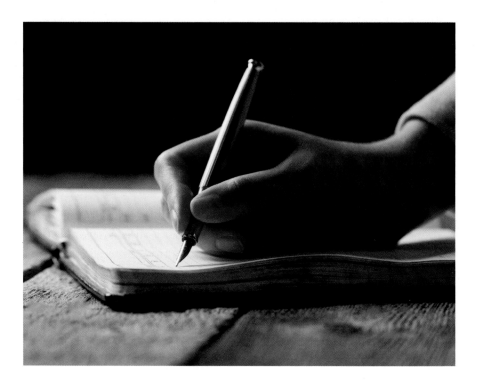

TAKE COPIOUS NOTES

Taking daily notes is essential for a variety of reasons. First and foremost, it is important to track signs and symptoms along the way, for yourself and your doctor, in order to gauge any progress or setbacks that may happen. Tracking daily (sometimes hourly) blood pressure, heart rate, and pulse is important in the process of determining whether or not you are or are optimized on thyroid hormones; it also may prove useful to your doctor and to you as a baseline for what is going on in your body when you are not feeling well. (It's also virtually impossible to rely on one's memory to retain daily or hourly vital statistics.)

I also believe keeping detailed notes can contribute to your relationship with any good doctor, because it shows you are willing, able, and serious enough to get to the bottom of the problem and solve it. Taking copious notes also exemplifies patient compliance and a high level of responsibility and accountability, which could inspire a doctor to take some risks with you when it comes to prescribing thyroid hormones.

On the other side of this point, I have brought some doctors a copy of my detailed notes on my daily/hourly vitals and symptomology, and they never even took a peek at it.

I would have never remembered exactly how I dosed myself on T3-only had I not taken notes (and I never thought I would use them in a book as an example), but I'm glad I did. You might not know in this moment how detailed notes may be useful in the future, but it is better to have them around in case you do need them.

TRACK VITALS

This one is tedious—I'm not going to lie. Especially if you have an office job or you are out of the house all day, because that means you will have to bring your thermometer and blood pressure device with you at all times and you'll have to take breaks during the day to track your vitals. Yes, it really is a pain. But in my case, I was willing to do everything I could to get better. If you want vibrant, optimal health badly enough, do everything that you can to succeed by keeping detailed records of your journey along the way.

SEEK A DOCTOR'S HELP

While this one didn't pan out for me during my first or second struggle with hypothyroidism, I do know people who found the right doctor during their early stages of hypothyroidism and were steered in the right direction by an informed physician. Even if you're in the same situation I was, where I had no choice but to take matters into my own hands I still kept searching for a doctor throughout the ordeal. Finally, I found Dr. Foresman, who is the most amazing doctor I have ever met. His invaluable contributions to my health have been life-saving, which is why I interviewed him for this book.

DON'T RELY SOLELY ON YOUR DOCTOR

No matter how awesome your doctor is, *you* are the one living in your body. We all need to take responsibility for our own health. You need to get copies of your lab results and study them, always. Learn about your body by learning about the blood tests and what they mean and what the optimal values are; we all have access to the internet. Just because something is *within range* on a blood test does not mean it's *optimal*.

Many years ago, my first doctor failed to notice that my ferritin (iron storage) was problematic because the result was *within range*, but very low in the range. A result of 30 in a range of 10–150 is anemia (a condition in which you don't have enough healthy red blood cells to carry adequate oxygen to the body's tissues) and can *cause* thyroid problems, but because there wasn't an "H" or "L" (for high or low) next to the result, the doctor didn't notice. That value of 30 continued to lower until it was at 10 and at the very bottom of the ferritin reference range of 10–150. I was indeed very anemic, and it could have been caught years earlier had the doctor understood the difference between *optimal* and *within range*. I initially made the mistake of trusting the first doctor I saw when he said, "Everything looks good. Your thyroid is fine." I believed him. Had I just combed through my blood results and done some internet research at the onset of my symptoms, I might have caught the low ferritin issue and the fact that I was incorrectly tested for hypothyroidism with the TSH test.

Double-check your doctor's work, because it's *your* body, and no one else is going to care about it more than you do. It is imperative that you take the ultimate responsibility for your health, and it starts with learning about whatever health issue you may have and investigating lab work. Some thyroid patients suffered for eight to twenty years because they trusted their health solely to their doctor. Continually search, seek, and never give up; you actually might have a better solution than your doctor! In my experience, perseverance prevails.

ADOPT A PALEO/PRIMAL LIFESTYLE

The most effective way of eating and living for healthy adrenal function, blood glucose management, weight loss/ideal body composition, brain function, and optimal thyroid hormone metabolism is the paleo/primal lifestyle. It also happens to be the only lifestyle aligned with our human genetics.

Thyroid Experts

As you try to optimize your thyroid medication, some issues may arise that your doctor might not anticipate or understand. But I lay them out for you in the next chapter, and you can become informed so you don't have to rely on outdated testing and ancient dosing strategies to achieve optimum health and happiness.

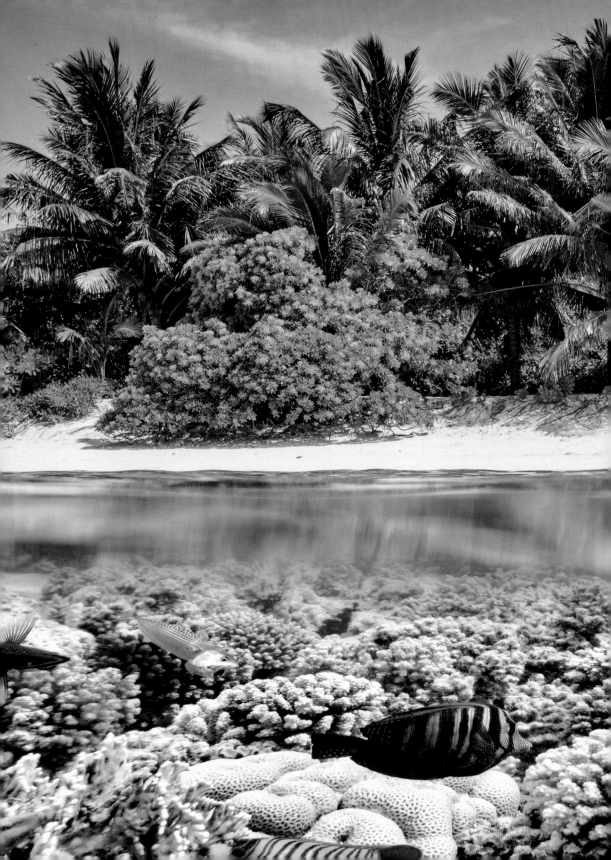

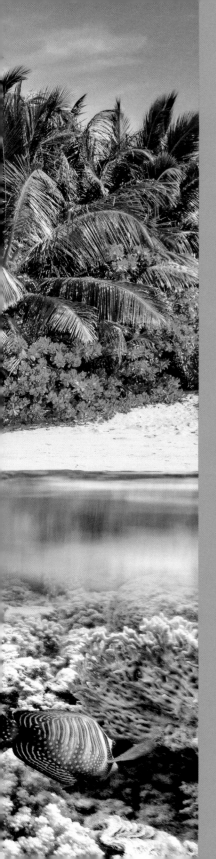

CHAPTER FOUR

Delving Deeper into T3 and Reverse T3

*As you will read in my personal story in chapter 8, I was doing well on NDT for many years, until I wasn't. I developed a severe Reverse T3 problem (a form of hypothyroidism), where the NDT no longer worked **for** me, but instead worked **against** me. Reverse T3 issues, the new hidden epidemic of hypothyroidism, are on the rise. I want you to be prepared if these issues ever surface for you.*

Reverse T3

Reverse T3 is a tricky business for a variety of reasons, of which the scariest is many doctors don't know what it is, and therefore they don't know how to test for it or fix it. As discussed, T4 is a prohormone that converts into the metabolically active thyroid hormone T3. Reverse T3 issues happen when, due to a variety of factors, the T4 converts into too much Reverse T3, *which is the inactive form of T3* (thus making the person hypothyroid). Hypothyroid symptoms show up despite the fact that Free T3 blood levels may look optimal or even high.

Imagine Reverse T3 like this: RT3 will guard and block the T3 cell receptor, preventing the T3 from getting into that cell to do its job and take you out of a hypothyroid state. Reverse T3 is actually your body's way of protecting you by lowering your metabolic rate in times of crisis, stress, inflammation, or disease. (Recall my description of it as your body's "alarm" on page 29.) Because T3 is a powerful energy-producer in the body, the body prefers to lower metabolic rate while it deals with other health issues. For example, in the case of chronic dieting, if one is over-restricting calories, the body thinks it is in a state of starvation and so the body will convert T4 into RT3 in an attempt to lower metabolic rate (fat-burning) because the body wants to hold onto the fat you currently have until you are out of "starvation" mode and can fuel the body with enough nutrition to turn off the RT3 alarm.

T4 to T3 conversion problems can be caused by a number of factors, including chronic stress, depression, starvation/extreme dieting, insulin resistance, diabetes, chronic fatigue syndrome, fibromyalgia, chronic inflammation, iron deficiency, exposure to toxins and heavy metals, low and/or high cortisol problems (adrenal dysfunction or fatigue).

Reverse T3 issues feel exactly like when you are hypothyroid—awful! During my Reverse T3 issue, I experienced the same symptoms as when I was seriously hypothyroid before getting optimized on NDT many years prior: exhaustion, depression, weight gain at a rapid rate (especially around the waist), brain fog, myxedema, a sense of being overwhelmed by small tasks, inability to think clearly, and extremely dry, cracked skin on my index finger. Luckily, I caught my RT3 problem much faster than my initial hypothyroid diagnosis nine years prior, so, thankfully, I did not end up experiencing all the symptoms I had suffered during my first bout of hypothyroidism.

Fixing Reverse T3 with Thyroid Hormones

- **Decreasing NDT dose/Adding T3:** Some people find success only by weaning off of T4-containing hormones and then starting direct T3-only. However, there are people who find success by either decreasing their NDT or adding T3 to their NDT dose. It can take anywhere from eight to twelve weeks to fully correct an RT3 problem.
- **Selenium/Milk Thistle/Liver Support:** Cleansing and supporting the liver is essential, because much of the RT3 is produced in the liver. Milk thistle is the standard go-to choice for liver support, but there are other, more complex, adrenal support options too. Low selenium levels can contribute to high RT3 levels. Making sure that your selenium intake is adequate can assist in correcting RT3 issues (see page 55 for more on selenium).
- **Addressing underlying culprits:** After one either decreases their NDT or starts on T3-only, the underlying causes of RT3 (infections, Lyme disease, low iron, insufficient adrenal function, and poor nutrition/lifestyle) need to be addressed. Adopting a paleo lifestyle promotes optimal absorption of nutrients and assists in healing fatigued adrenals, while also balancing blood sugar levels.

WEANING OFF T4 AND STARTING T3-ONLY

Since people with RT3 issues who take thyroid hormones are usually on a T4-containing hormone (only T4 converts into RT3), some people slowly wean themselves off their T4-containing hormone over a few weeks. Some just stop taking it cold turkey and wait seven to ten days before starting T3-only. The philosophy is that the T4 has a half-life of about a week, so it will take that amount of time to decrease the T4 before introducing T3. The dosage values are different, depending on the kind/form of T3. I use 25 mcg pills (that can be taken sublingually) and a pill cutter (sometimes my teeth when I'm in a jam). With 25 mcg pills, you can accurately break or cut them into 6.25 mcg and 12.5 mcg doses.

DOSING DIRECT T3 (NOT SUSTAINED-RELEASE T3)

There is no compelling evidence that suggests T4 is necessary to human health and longevity, yet naysayers claim T4 is essential for brain function and healthy hair. As I described in chapter 3, *multi-dosing* is key with direct T3 due to its fast-acting nature. The half-life of T3 is short, but it is a powerful hormone. T3 is usually taken in three to five divided doses per day. Doses can be anywhere from three to seven hours apart. Timing of the doses is based on when symptoms tell you it's time for more (like feeling exhausted to the onset of a higher heart rate). Usually when you feel exhaustion or depression set in, those could be indications that you needed a T3 dose thirty to sixty minutes prior to those symptoms.

Foundations for Taking T3

STABLE TEMPERATURES

Stable temperature *averages* indicate adrenal sufficiency, meaning the adrenals are functioning properly. The ideal is five days' worth of temperatures that vary no more than 0.2°F or 0.1°C. Temperatures might decrease or be erratic after each T3 increase; therefore, people on T3 consider it helpful to have five days of stable temperatures *before* increasing T3.

This temperature-taking protocol is different than taking your basal and afternoon temperatures as previously discussed in chapter 2.

Thyroid hormones need cortisol (an adrenal hormone) in order to work in the cells, so a decline in cortisol production reduces the metabolism of thyroid hormones, which then places more pressure on the adrenal glands to produce more cortisol. This loop can push you down a spiral staircase into more adrenal issues. Some scientists believe that the entrance of thyroid hormones into the cells is delegated by adrenal hormones. (More on adrenals and cortisol in chapter 6.)

TEMPERATURE-TAKING PROTOCOL FOR ADRENAL SUFFICIENCY

Use an old-school mercury thermometer or a Geratherm thermometer (digital thermometers are unreliable).

Sit quietly for at least fifteen minutes before taking your temperature.

Don't eat, drink, smoke, exercise, during this time (and preferably not for thirty minutes prior).

Sit comfortably and put the thermometer under your tongue for a solid seven to ten minutes.

Remove the thermometer and record your temperature.

Take your temperature three times a day:

First temperature three hours after waking.

Second temperature six hours after waking.

Third temperature nine hours after waking.

Average the three temperatures and round to one decimal.

Example

Day 1

Wake up 7:00 a.m.

Temperature 1: 10:00 a.m. = 97.8°F

Temperature 2: 1:00 p.m. = 98.1°F

Temperature 3: 4:00 p.m. = 98.3°F

Add the temperatures together = 294.2

Divide by 3 = 98.06 (rounded to 98.1)

Final value for Day 1 = 98.1°F

After you have calculated the final value for each of the five days, you can assess the variation among them to determine adrenal sufficiency for T3 dosing.

ELEVATED TEMPERATURES

Hypothyroidism classically results in low body temperature (impaired metabolism). But temperatures can be falsely elevated due to the following issues: Low iron, low sodium, high cortisol, low aldosterone, high progesterone, and infections. The menstrual cycle can also change the level of temperature *but not its stability*. Increased progesterone after ovulation can increase temperature to 99ºF.

IRON INSUFFICIENCY

In the presence of insufficient iron, T3 can cause anxiety. One can stop taking T3 until iron levels improve, or one can reduce the dose of T3 while simultaneously working to raise iron levels.

Dosing T3

The first plan of attack should be to assess, treat, and fix the underlying causes of RT3 issues, and then see whether or not the conversion of T4 to T3 starts to kick in again. In my case, addressing the underlying causes of faulty T4 to T3 conversion did not work. In this scenario, taking the thyroid hormone T3 or "T3-only" (without any T4) is the ultimate answer for seemingly uncorrectable conversion issues. Think about it: if the whole point of having a thyroid is so that you can get adequate levels of T3 into your body, then if someone's T4 is not converting to T3 (whether they take T4 orally or whether their own thyroid gland releases T4 naturally), you have to give the person what they're not getting! Which is T3.

Inadequate T3 levels will spiral daily life into a living nightmare riddled with health issues. Taking T3 directly, without any T4, eliminates any potential conversion issues and resolves Reverse T3 issues undeniably, because T3 on its own does not convert into Reverse T3. I recognize that the natural way our thyroid glands are meant to work is by dispensing a lot of T4, a little bit of T3, and then converting a big chunk of T4 into T3. And I still believe that mimicry of our natural system should certainly be the first protocol of thyroid treatment attempted. I am in no way favoring T3-only as the first choice of thyroid hormone replacement for hypothyroid patients. However, with a growing number of patients experiencing Reverse T3 issues, the medical community needs to recognize T3-only treatment as valid.

Everyone should work with a doctor on treating a Reverse T3 issue, but I didn't get that opportunity, like many fellow RT3 sufferers. Below are my T3-only dosing notes for the month of April 2012, when I started T3-only. I dosed myself with T3 after I was off NDT completely for an entire month. I was hoping that my own thyroid gland would kick back into gear, but after a month off NDT I was extremely hypothyroid; my Free T3 and Free T4 were at the bottom of the ranges.

Hopefully, this dosing example can provide doctors and patients with a snapshot of how someone can successfully and conservatively dose direct T3. Common starting doses of T3 are between 5 mcg and 10 mcg (some T3 brands come in 5 mcg pills). I used 25 mcg pills. A common starting dose of T3 for people using 25 mcg pills is between 6.25– and 12.5 mcg. I also tracked my blood pressure, pulse, and temperature – four to five times a day during this time.

DATE	DOSAGE AND NOTES
4/2	Start T3! 6.25 mcg@7:00 a.m.
4/3	12.5 mcg @7:00 a.m.
4/4	12.5 mcg @7:00 a.m.
4/5	12.5 mcg @7:00 a.m. / 12.5 mcg@4:00 p.m. (Afternoon dose felt like "too much.")
4/6	12.5 mcg @7:00 a.m. (Dropped yesterday's 4:00 p.m. dose.)
4/7	Decide to split the 12.5 mcg into two doses because the 12.5 mcg felt like too much to handle at once: 6.25 mcg@7:00 a.m. & 6.25 mcg@5:00 p.m. (Dry cracked skin on my finger is gone today! Noticeable weight/bloat "deflation.")

DATE	DOSAGE AND NOTES
4/8	6.25 mcg@7:00 a.m. & 6.25 mcg@5:00 p.m.
4/9	6.25 mcg@7:00 a.m. & 6.25 mcg@5:00 p.m.
4/11	Added third dose midday: 6.25 mcg@7:00 a.m., 6.25 mcg@12:00 p.m., 6.25 mcg@4:00 p.m.
4/12	6.25 mcg@7:00 a.m., 6.25 mcg@12:00 p.m., 6.25 mcg@4:00 p.m.
4/13	6.25 mcg@7:00 a.m., 6.25 mcg@12:00 p.m., 6.25 mcg@4:00 p.m. (Feeling much better!)
4/14	Added fourth evening dose: 6.25 mcg@7:00 a.m., 6.25 mcg@12:00 p.m., 6.25 mcg@4:00 p.m., 6.25 mcg@9:00 p.m.
4/15	6.25 mcg@7:00 a.m., 6.25 mcg@12:00 p.m., 6.25 mcg@4:00 p.m. / 6.25 mcg@9:00 p.m.
4/16	Increase morning dose to 12.5 mcg: 12.5 mcg@7:00 a.m., 6.25 mcg@12:00p.m., 6.25 mcg@4:00 p.m., 6.25 mcg@9:00 p.m.
4/17	12.5 mcg@7:00 a.m., 6.25 mcg@12:00 p.m., 6.25 mcg@4:00 p.m., 6.25 mcg@9:00 p.m.
4/18	12.5 mcg@7:00 a.m., 6.25 mcg@12:00 p.m., 6.25 mcg@4:00 p.m., 6.25 mcg@9:00 p.m.
4/19	Increase 12:00 p.m. doses to 12.5 mcg: 12.5 mcg@7:00 a.m., 12.5 mcg@12:00 p.m., 6.25 mcg@4:00 p.m., 6.25 mcg@9:00 p.m. (After increasing the 12:00 p.m. dose, the whole day was energy-filled, mental clarity, feeling positive. Noticed a tiny headache but went away after a couple of hours.)
4/20	Same dosing above. Fell asleep much easier than previous few days where I tossed and turned for a while before getting to sleep.
4/21	Same dosing above. Felt great energy from early morning on…all day.

DATE	DOSAGE AND NOTES
4/22	Same dosing as above.
4/23	Increased third dose to 12.5 mcg: 12.5 mcg@7:00 a.m., 12.5 mcg@12:00 p.m., 12.5 mcg@4:00 p.m., 6.25 mcg@9:00 p.m.
4/24	Moved the second dose to 11:30 a.m. instead of 12:00 p.m. Starting to drop in energy big time at 12:00 p.m. so I moved second dose to 11:30 a.m., 12.5mcg: 12.5 mcg@7:00 a.m., 12.5 mcg@11:30 a.m., 12.5 mcg@4:00 p.m., 6.25 mcg@9:00 p.m.
4/25	Same dosing as above, feeling good. 100x better than when I started T3!
4/26	Increased fourth dose to 12.5 mcg: 12.5 mcg@7:00 a.m., 12.5 mcg@11:30 a.m., 12.5 mcg@4:00 p.m., 12.5 mcg@9:00 p.m. (50 mcg of T3 total per day)
4/27–4/29	Same dosing as above.
4/30	Increase morning dose to 18.75 mcg: 18.75 mcg@7:00 a.m., 12.5 mcg@11:30 a.m., 12.5 mcg@4:00 p.m., 12.5 mcg@9:00 p.m. (56.25 mcg T3 per day)

After April 2012, I eventually increased to 100 mcg of T3 per day, split into evenly divided doses of 25 mcg. That worked for a while, but shortly after adopting a paleo lifestyle, the 100 mcg of T3 per day made me *hyper*thyroid (high temperatures, high pulse, anxiousness, restlessness, sweating, etc.). Likely, the paleo lifestyle I had adopted had balanced my blood sugar levels, began correcting insulin resistance, and balanced my adrenals, which all led to more efficient thyroid hormone metabolism.

Over the course of the three and a half years I have been on T3-only, I have made a few adjustments. I am always on alert for the signs and symptoms that I might need to lower or increase my dose. In my experience thus far, those dosage adjustments range between 6.25 mcg and 12.5 mcg.

MY CURRENT T3 DOSING SCHEDULE: 56.25 MCG OF T3 PER DAY

TIME	DOSAGE
5:45/6:00 a.m.	25 mcg
11:00 a.m.	18.75 mcg
4:00 p.m.	6.25 mcg
10:00/10:30 p.m.	6.25 mcg

Some people on T3-only adopt an evenly divided dosing schedule. I eventually adopted a *tailored-dose strategy*. I found that my body and brain needed more T3 in the first half of the day than the last half of the day. This is all individual. Some patients cannot tolerate nighttime doses of T3, yet I have never had an issue with this. Finding the right combination of dosage and dosing times is a personal experimentation process and everyone has different needs. Sometimes I take my second dose thirty minutes later than usual, depending on how I feel. Over time, I have developed an intuitive sense about T3 dosing.

Sometimes I need a little less T3 for seasonal or other reasons. To be consistent with my dosing times, I program recurring alarms on my iPhone. I also adjust my dosing times if my wake/sleep hours change significantly (although I usually keep consistent sleep/wake times). I always carry T3 with me when I leave the house. I have a pill-holder keychain so that my T3 is always with my car/house keys. When I travel, I give a relative *and* a friend each a package of T3, so in the event I am somewhere in the world and lose my medication or it gets stolen, my friend or family member can FedEx it to me. As an emergency back-up, I also travel with a bottle of NDT in case something happens to my T3 and I cannot quickly acquire it.

What Does T3-Only Feel Like?

It feels as though I was never hypothyroid to begin with! For me, T3-only feels more consistent than NDT did. I am open to the idea of one day attempting to go back on NDT as an experiment to see if I can convert T4 to T3 properly and see if NDT works for me as well as T3-only does.

There are stories of patients who went back on NDT and found that it worked better for them and felt *smoother* than T3. Others claim that going back on NDT did not work for them, so they went back on T3. But two hours after taking my first dose of T3-only, I felt like a miracle had occurred. I immediately felt my brain wake up, and I suddenly had a level of mental focus that had not been there months prior. My depression lifted and in that moment I knew that T3 would solve my RT3 problem—and it did.

It's tough to think about going back on a substance (T4) that I am not positive will consistently convert to the T3 levels that I need on a daily basis, because it failed me once before. By taking direct T3 I have eliminated a very problematic middleman. Every time I put direct T3 into my mouth, I am certain that it's going to do its job, because it requires zero conversion. That said, dosing NDT is much easier, widely available, and easy to get a prescription for. I will try going back on NDT at some point in the future.

Will I Be on the Same T3 Dose and Dosing Schedule Forever?

*Dosages and dosing schedules are individual and change with how your body processes T3. My T3 dosages have changed over time, yet my **dosing schedule** has mostly remained the same. Some patients say that after a substantial amount of time on T3, they were able to move down to three doses per day versus five doses per day. It's important to track vitals and symptoms and follow your intuition.*

Blood Tests Values on T3

Most of the time, people who are optimized on T3-only (direct T3) will see the following on lab results:

TSH will be suppressed.

Free T4 will be suppressed.

Free T3 could be anywhere from the top of the range to 10–20% over the top of the range.

Free T3 levels are individual, and as long as the patient is not hyperthyroid, *blood values do not alone define hyperthyroidism.* Hyperthyroidism caused by excess T3 consumption is easily assessed through tracking temperature, blood pressure, pulse, and signs/symptoms of overstimulation.

I grew up in downtown Chicago and I am a fast-speaking individual. While on T3-only, I had a doctor tell me she thought I was hyperthyroid because I "seemed overstimulated based on how fast I was talking." First of all, everyone who knows me, including my parents, would laugh at this, because I've talked fast my entire life. Furthermore, I think we can all agree the word "seem" is not a medical diagnosis. I'd like doctors to start testing/tracking a patient's vitals to see if the patient is truly hyperthyroid, versus *assuming* that a patient is hyperthyroid based on talking speed combined with higher Free T3 blood levels. This same doctor also told me that she could lose her medical license if she prescribed the amount of T3 I was taking, and she told me that I was basically killing myself. That said, my physical exam and blood work taken by this doctor reflected great health along with stellar EKG results, so I find her *guesstimate* interesting and full of holes. Needless to say, I didn't return to that doctor!

Using T3-Only Without a Doctor

Not one doctor I contacted was willing to prescribe T3-only to help me correct my Reverse T3 issue. Even though it was a scary position to be in, I had to trust myself. I had resolved my first bout of hypothyroidism on my own using NDT, and I was confident and determined to fix my RT3 problem too. I was extremely diligent, aware, conservative, and responsible with how I approached dosing myself with both NDT, and years later, with T3. In both scenarios I found thyroid hormones without a prescription.

I would never suggest that anyone attempt to fix a thyroid problem on their own, without a doctor's guidance, but I did not have such an opportunity. And there are many patients out there like me, who have come up against one uninformed doctor after another and continue to get sicker and sicker with every day that passes. What are people like us supposed to do? The state of thyroid health care has to change!

T3 and NDT Dose Comparison

One grain (or 60 mg) of desiccated thyroid (NDT) equals about 25 mcg of T3. If someone was previously optimized on 3 grains (~180 mg) of desiccated thyroid before they developed a Reverse T3 problem, 75 mcg of T3-only might be their optimal dose (sometimes higher or lower).

My current optimal T3 dose is 56.25 mcg per day (which equates to roughly 2¼ grains of NDT). Yet, when I was optimized on NDT for many years prior, I consistently felt best between 3 and 3.5 grains, which equates to about 75 mcg of T3. However, I was not living a paleo/primal lifestyle during my years on NDT.

After going paleo, I was able to lower my dosage of T3 *by half*, likely the result of optimal blood glucose management, healthy adrenals, and optimal thyroid hormone metabolism, which a paleo/primal lifestyle promotes.

Why Multi-dosing T3 Is a Game-Changer

One might think that taking 56.25 mcg of T3 in a once-daily dose would do the trick, but there are a variety of nuances that make a single T3 dose of 56.25 mcg or more a poor strategy. T3 reaches 95% saturation in all of the tissues within four hours, so dosing T3 once a day doesn't make a lot of sense, and it could be harmful. Due to the short-lived rise and fall of T3, a single large dose could cause an unnecessarily elevated heart rate and negatively affect heart health, along with over-stimulation symptoms. A 50 mcg or 75 mcg dose could be too much for someone to handle all at once.

This is what the pharmaceutical company Pfizer has to say about dosing T3 in their "Physician Prescribing Information" PDF on Cytomel (T3) (at labeling.pfizer.com/ShowLabeling.aspx?id=703):

> Recommended starting dosage is 25 mcg daily. Daily dosage then may be increased by up to 25 mcg every 1 or 2 weeks. Usual maintenance dose is 25 to75 mcg daily. The rapid onset and dissipation of action of liothyronine sodium (T3), as compared with levothyroxine sodium (T4), has led some clinicians to prefer its use in patients who might be more susceptible to the untoward effects of thyroid medication. **However, the wide swings in serum T3 levels that follow its administration and the possibility of more pronounced cardiovascular side effects tend to counterbalance the stated advantages.** Cytomel (liothyronine sodium) Tablets…may also be preferred when impairment of peripheral conversion of T4 to T3 is suspected.

The sentence that I bolded, above, makes me laugh whenever I read it. When Pfizer states that the cardiac risks to taking T3-only might outweigh the benefits, presumably, they are not factoring in the protocol of *multi-dosing*. I guess dosing T3 more than once or twice a day didn't factor into their literature! A common practice among people on T3-only (direct T3, not sustained-release) is to dose three to five times per day and usually in increments of *25 mcg or less per dose*. Multi-dosing T3 needs to be considered in Pfizer's Cytomel literature for physicians, and doctors need to strongly consider the benefits of multi-dosing patients with direct T3 in this way, instead of solely relying on sustained-release T3 as the "only T3 option" available to patients who cannot tolerate T4 or convert T4.

Why Use T3 to Fix Reverse T3

There are other ways to fix a Reverse T3 problem, but T3-only is more of a sure bet, and often people choose the direct route to success. I tried every other option first, and T3-only was the only protocol that worked for me. The idea behind why T3-only successfully treats an RT3 problem is this: when T4 converts into RT3, the RT3 essentially blocks the T3 receptors, causing T3 to pool in the bloodstream, and then T3 cannot enter the cell to do its job. This is why people feel hypothyroid when they have a Reverse T3 problem, even though they are taking T4-only or T4/T3 combination thyroid hormone replacement. This is also why a Free T3 test can look optimal, or even high, on a lab result, even though the hypothyroid person isn't getting the metabolic benefits of T3.

The key is to clear out all the excess T4 in the body so that it can no longer convert into RT3, which is causing the problem in the first place. Only T4 converts into RT3; T3 does not make RT3. It can take between eight and twelve weeks before you start to feel well and until the T3 finally gets out of the parking lot, into the office, and punches in to work (because production of RT3 dissipated and RT3 finally stopped blocking the T3 receptor). For me, it took about ten weeks after starting on T3 to feel *major* symptom relief, but I felt some relief in just hours after my first T3 dose.

T3: The Primal Perspective

T3 is a metabolic powerhouse responsible for fat burning. Aside from getting rid of excess T4 in the body, Reverse T3 exists to protect us from increasing metabolism in stressful situations. Perceived stress can stem from nutrient deficiencies, inadequate caloric intake, chronic exercising, blood sugar imbalances, infections, and adrenal issues. Take a chronic dieter who overexercises: their primal DNA blueprint interprets the stress along these lines, "We are not going to give this person any more fat-burning metabolism-causing T3 because this person can't handle it right now. They must be running from danger (adrenals are all over the place and blood sugar spikes are common). They are starving, so we are not going to give them a powerful fat-burning hormone in an environment where they need extra fat reserves in order to survive. Oh, and by the way, we're also going to lower levels of sex hormones and decrease libido so that they won't want to (or can't) procreate right now, because clearly they're in no position to bring a child into this world when they can barely feed themselves and are busy fleeing from danger."

On a personal note, hypothyroidism showed up in my life when I was living a low-fat, low-carbohydrate, chronic cardio existence. It is painfully ironic that in my quest and dedication to achieve the ultimate level of health and fitness I was led down a path to a debilitating condition, which monopolized five to six years of my life and made me fat, depressed, and very sick.

- -

RT3 and Stressors

If you are an athlete engaged in excessive running, your body interprets that as a stress and assumes you are in danger. So it's going to respond by helping you keep your fat reserves until perceived danger goes away. If you are living a low-fat, high-carbohydrate existence (or low-fat/low-carbohydrate) and chronically doing cardio exercise on top of having very low body fat and low weight, then your body thinks you're starving and stressed and it's not going to let you burn the very little fat you have left on your body until it senses the perceived danger is clear. Hence, people who overtrain, who chronically limit caloric intake, or have a lot of stress in their lives are susceptible to Reverse T3 issues. The diet and lifestyle aspects of the Paleo Thyroid Solution have a critical role in RT3, as we shall see.

- -

Common Factors Preventing the Conversion of T4 to T3

- **Mineral deficiencies:** Low levels of selenium, zinc, iron, and B12.
- **Liver issues:** Compromised liver function affects the conversion of T4 to T3. The liver is continually converting T4 to RT3 in order to get rid of unused/excess T4. When your body needs to buckle down, conserve energy, and focus on other things, more of the T4 can get converted into RT3, and the T3 will get lower and lower.
- **Adrenal problems:** High and/or low cortisol.
- **Gastrointestinal issues:** Gut issues can cause problems with the absorption of minerals, which can lead to low nutrient levels that might ignite an RT3 problem. Even if you don't have deficiencies in selenium or zinc, suboptimal digestion or more serious conditions like leaky gut syndrome, candida infections, or IBS can all contribute to low T3 levels. Inflammation in the gut can reduce T3 by raising levels of cortisol, which can contribute to more RT3 production.
- **Stress:** Physical and mental stress can trigger the body into protection mode and set off the body's natural emergency alarm, Reverse T3.

T3 and the Brain

Brain cells have more T3 receptors than any other tissues, and adequate amounts of T3 (whether through conversion or direct T3 dosing) are critical to proper brain function and the development of both newborns' and adults' brains. Optimizing thyroid hormone metabolism is critical to normal brain function. Untreated hypothyroidism in adults is associated with cognitive defects along with balance and motor skill issues. Thyroid disorders have been closely linked to psychiatric disorders, and patients are often misdiagnosed with depression or bipolar disorder without understanding that one of the causes can be low levels of T3. Patients diagnosed with depression, anxiety, or bipolar disorder should be tested by doctors for thyroid issues in order to determine whether the cause is inadequate levels of T3 (or too much T3).

T3 thyroid hormone is used for treating depression! T3 interacts with brain receptors and crafts the brain's sensitivity to neurotransmitters involved with memory, alertness, focus, emotions, and disposition. Given how crucial T3 is to every aspect of our lives, it makes sense why a person on T4-only, who is only having their Free T4 and TSH tested by their endocrinologist, could be headed down a dangerous path. Many patients, on T4-only, get misdiagnosed with depression and prescribed antidepressants, because no one is testing their Free T3 levels to see if their T4 is converting into adequate levels of T3. It is essential to test Free T3 levels, regardless of the type of thyroid hormone replacement used.

On T3-only, I experience a very sharp sense of how T3 is affecting my brain and body. I've experienced my brain on extremely low levels of T3, too much T3, and almost but not quite enough T3. I can feel the difference of a 6.25 mcg subtraction or addition to my daily dosing of T3. When I had extremely low levels of T3 I could barely think, I was very depressed, and it was an awful mind to live in. It felt like my brain was in a fog, similar to having a stuffy head and all you can do is stare into space, and nothing seemed like fun. Other symptoms include impaired memory, inability to focus, and a sense of being paralyzed in

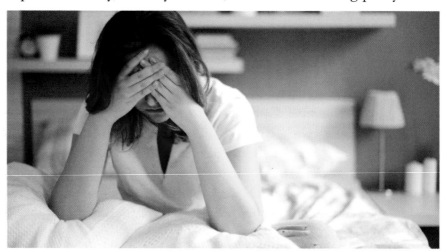

terms of motivation. I continually thought to myself, "What the hell is wrong with me?" I felt as if I was completely aware of my lack of motivation, but I still couldn't seem to do anything about it. What I have noticed in comparing lab work to symptoms is that if my Free T3 drops to a certain level, I inevitably become depressed, overwhelmed, unfocused, unmotivated, and other cognitive issues arise, such as saying words incorrectly or jumbling up their pronunciation.

"T3 is found in large quantities in the limbic system of the brain, the area that is important for emotions such as joy, panic, anger, and fear. If you don't have enough T3, or if its action is blocked, an entire cascade of neurotransmitter abnormalities may ensue and can lead to mood and energy changes, including depression. Hypothyroidism and depression are related on many levels. The main building block for the neurotransmitter serotonin and for thyroid hormone (both T3 and T4) is the amino acid tryptophan, the same amino acid needed for the neurotransmitter norepinephrine, which stabilizes mood and anxiety. This means it is quite possible that low thyroid function can deplete your body of serotonin and other mood-stabilizing neurotransmitters. It also means that chronic depression and sadness may deplete your body of tyrosine stores and T3, which is also necessary to maintain healthy mood and energy."

—Christiane Northrup, MD, drnorthrup.com

Too Much T3

Too much T3 can have the opposite effect on the brain. When I was on too much T3 and hyperthyroid, it I felt as if I was in a state of hyper focus, which at first glance might seem desirable; who wouldn't want to be super focused, motivated and energized, right? Wrong! I am already a highly focused and motivated person, so hyperthyroidism felt like being on heavy amounts of speed. The initial surge of energy ultimately does not last, and eventually exhaustion creeps in due to hyperthyroid effects on adrenals and blood sugar imbalances, and so on.

Other disadvantages I experienced of too much T3 were an overall sense of detachment from people and the outside world; I felt as if I didn't have the patience to communicate because my brain was working too fast and functioning on such a different level that I couldn't relate to people, nor did I want to be around them. My body temperature was too high; I was too warm all the time. (Whereas with hypothyroidism, people often experience a drop in body temperature, and feel cold all the time.) Other symptoms showed up like increased heart rate, anxiety, increased appetite, reaching my maximum heart rate too quickly and feeling out of breath and weak when walking uphill. I experienced nerve pain in my hip region and had increased muscle soreness all over my body (something I also experienced with low levels of T3). When I was hyperthyroid, upon waking in the morning, I would bolt out of bed with restless energy, because I just couldn't lay still for thirty seconds after the alarm went off. After I lowered my T3 dose and I became normal again, I finally enjoyed the luxury of slowly waking up in the morning and starting the day in a relaxed manner.

Thyroid hormone management is akin to the story of Goldilocks: the porridge needs to be not too hot, not too cold, but just right.

T3 and the Heart

T3 plays a very important role not only in normalizing cholesterol levels, but also in affecting healthy blood pressure and a healthy heart rate. Low levels of T3 can go hand in hand with a poorly functioning heart rate, increased blood pressure, and hardening of the arteries.

I have had ideal cholesterol labs my entire life, except for when I was hypothyroid. After becoming optimized on thyroid hormone replacement and reaching optimal levels of T3, all my cholesterol labs returned to being optimal.

When seeing a doctor for problems related to the heart or the liver or for cholesterol, you should ask your doctor to test thyroid function as well.

Good News

I know that optimizing your medication, especially if you have RT3 issues, can feel complicated and overwhelming. The good news is that we're about to get to the fun part: delicious food, fun activity, lots of sleep, and less stress.

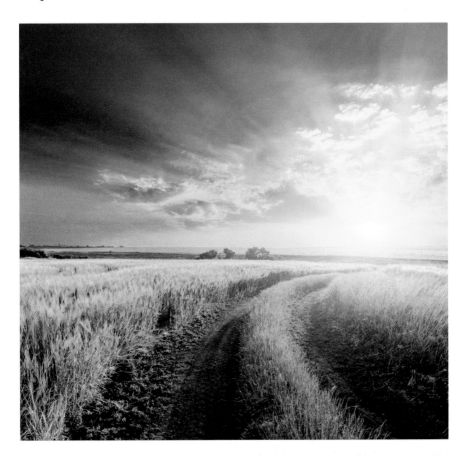

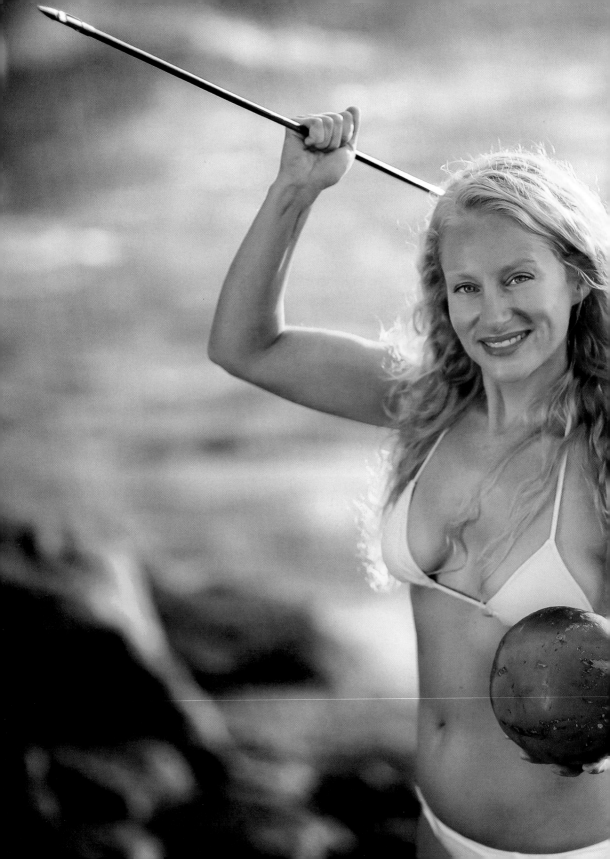

Paleo/Primal Eating and Exercise

*As humans, we are all born with a
DNA map to health and happiness.
In fact, every species was born with
their own DNA maps. Unfortunately,
over the past 10,000 years humans have
thrown away that map and unknowingly
taken a detour in the wrong direction,
which opened the door and invited in
the diseases of modern life.*

PALEO THYROID SOLUTION PRINCIPLES

- Eat plants, animals, fish, and fat.

- Eliminate grains, beans, and legumes.

- Limit dairy and potatoes to *very occasional* consumption (unless you're an athlete).

- Stay under 150 total carbohydrates per day (smaller women, like me, might require 100 carbohydrates or less per day).

- Consume probiotics.

- Get adequate sleep.

- Manage stress.

- Stick with low-intensity exercise between 55% and 75% of your maximum heart rate.

- Do a fifteen-minute sprint session every seven to ten days (only if your hypothyroid symptoms are gone, and you have the adrenal strength to support a sprint session).

- Supplement/Optimize: vitamin D, omega-3 fatty acids, selenium, B12, iron, DHEA, vitamin C, magnesium, and sea salt (sea salt supports adrenal health).

- Only eat when you're hungry.

Why Paleo?

Ever since paleo became a popular buzz word, people have been grossly misinterpreting it on a variety of levels. Paleo, primal, ancestral, and evolutionary health are all terms that describe the same movement. The biggest misconception about a paleo lifestyle is that it is merely a list of foods you can or cannot eat. This could not be further from the truth. The paleo/primal lifestyle is different from any other eating strategy out there today. It enables you to get off the carbohydrate-dependency hamster wheel, which is the cause of so many diseases, and allows you to transition into a fat-burning machine.

WHAT IS A SUGAR-BURNER?

If you are a sugar-burner, your body is dependent on (i.e., addicted to) fueling itself on glucose. If you are a sugar-burner, you trained your body to function this way; many people do this unwittingly based on flawed, conventional diet wisdom that instructs people to eat every two to three hours and/or adopt a low-fat/high-carbohydrate diet. The reason so many people cannot lose weight or maintain weight loss without struggling is that they are sugar-burners.

You are a sugar-burner if:
- You cannot go more than eight-plus waking hours without eating because you will get cranky, have a drop in physical or mental energy, or experience other negative symptoms.
- You have hypoglycemia.
- You struggle to lose weight.
- You struggle to keep weight off.
- You cannot get food off of your mind, and you have food obsessions/addictions.
- You crave sugary foods, and it takes a ton of willpower to refuse the cravings.
- You crave grain-based carbohydrates like bread, rice, cereal, and baked goods/treats.
- You can't seem to burn fat.

- You are hungry every two to five hours.
- You have drops in energy during the day.

(Notice that a lot of the symptoms here are similar to what you experience when you are hypothyroid. Coincidence? Probably not.)

I used to be royally *obsessed* with food. At one point I thought about joining Overeaters Anonymous because I didn't understand why I was so food-obsessed. I couldn't go more than three to four hours without eating, or I would get very cranky and feel exhausted and mentally drained. Like many people, I thought the "eat every two to three hours" philosophy was the healthiest eating strategy, based on the information I read in almost every diet book on the market. And it certainly seemed in line with the symptoms I had when I did not follow that routine, so I believed the strategy had merit. However, at the time I didn't realize that there was a much easier and healthier way: *eating the way our bodies were genetically programmed to operate.*

WHAT IS A FAT-BURNER?

If you are a fat-burner, you can use the fat from your diet and the fat stored in your body to fuel yourself.

Fat has been the primary fuel source for humans for 2.5 million years, both from storage and as the predominant macronutrient in the human diet. In fact, it was the energy-rich, high-fat elements of animal products (particularly omega-3 fatty acids) that facilitated the development of a more complex brain and allowed humans to branch out from their predominantly vegetarian ape cousins to eventually rise to the top of the food chain.

Our genetic makeup is still the same as our hunter-gatherer ancestors who lived 50,000 years ago. Our bodies were genetically designed to burn fat, not glucose, as fuel.

Our bodies were genetically designed to burn fat, not glucose, as fuel.

Our preference for fat-burning conflicts with the government food pyramid, which suggests that carbohydrates should form the foundation of a healthy diet. The government food pyramid recommends eating six to eleven servings of grains per day and two to four servings of fruit, along with limiting fat intake and other irrational suggestions that lead to health issues. Our modern high-carbohydrate, grain-based diet has sparked a dependency on external carbohydrates for energy at the expense of efficient fat metabolism.

We are the only living things on the face of the Earth who have "food issues." Animals in the wild don't require food every two to three hours to maintain energy and stamina. Humans have burned fat as their primary source of energy throughout human evolution. Our hunter-gatherer ancestors were not only lean and fit, but they did not have diseases of modern life, such as type 2 diabetes, hypothyroidism, and autoimmune disorders, until the abrupt transition to a grain-based diet. The agricultural movement, and the decline of human health, entered the picture ten thousand years ago, once humans settled down in one area, stopped wandering, and started to domesticate animals. Dairy came on the scene about seven thousand years ago, and sugar showed up only two hundred years ago.

A high-carbohydrate, high-insulin-producing diet inhibits fat metabolism, making you dependent upon regular carbohydrate feedings in order to sustain mental and physical energy. (Read more about insulin on page 111.) This promotes a lifelong accumulation of excess body fat, an exhaustion of your adrenal glands' fight-or-flight stress responses, along with emotional tribulations related to eating. Living life as a sugar-burner is a never-ending struggle to balance calories in with calories out. A grain-infused, high-carbohydrate diet also promotes inflammation and free radical damage in the body, accelerating the aging process and contributing to all health problems, including heart disease and cancer.

Our hunter-gatherer ancestors ate a diet high in animal flesh and animal fat along with *very low-carbohydrate/low-sugar* consumption. Did you know that humans can live their entire lives without ever eating a single carbohydrate, but we could not survive without protein and fat? Not only will our bodies produce glucose on their own, but excess protein goes through a process called gluconeogenesis, which converts excess protein into glucose. So in times of overeating animal flesh in the wild, human bodies would turn that excess protein into carbohydrates.

We were all born with a perfect genetic formula to live long, happy lives and spend our time in lean, fit bodies with an abundance of mental and physical energy. The introduction of grains, sugar, dairy, and excess carbohydrate consumption has, over time, turned millions of people into sugar-burners who are glucose dependent. A sugar-burning existence will put you at risk for developing food addictions, hypoglycemia, insulin resistance, type 2 diabetes, and adrenal gland issues, all of which negatively affect thyroid hormone metabolism.

You are a fat-burner if:
- You can go more than eight to ten, even twenty-four hours without eating food *and still maintain incredible physical/mental energy and stamina with zero desire for food.*
- You effortlessly lose weight and maintain weight loss without mental or physical struggles.
- You "forget" about food and are not obsessed with your next meal.
- You don't crave sugar or grain-based foods.

Like our hunter-gatherer ancestors, a person who is fat adapted can go eight to twenty-four hours without eating and still have full mental focus and physical energy. When is the last time you went more than five hours without food and didn't have a meltdown? It is rare for millions of Americans. Continuing to live as a sugar-burner will contribute to unhealthy adrenal function, poor glucose management and can even lead to insulin resistance and type 2 diabetes. Furthermore, the consumption of grains can lead to nutrient deficiencies and can cause/ignite autoimmune disorders such as Hashimoto's, arthritis, and more.

However, when people adopt a paleo lifestyle correctly, they experience a freedom that only fat-burners understand. Being fat adapted is an amazing and wonderful life that I wish I had known about over a decade ago.

Did Our Hunter-Gatherer Ancestors Have Hypothyroidism?

Based on the Paleolithic eating and lifestyle habits of our hunter-gatherer ancestors, it's highly doubtful they had hypothyroidism. The earliest mention of thyroid issues dates back to around 12,000 years ago in China. Coincidentally, wheat and barley were introduced to China from the Middle East during that time, reflected in the name of the mythical Chinese emperor "Emperor of the Five Grains." I will go into depth later in this chapter as to why grains are toxic and need to be eliminated from our diets in order to achieve optimal thyroid health and metabolism; however, suffice to say for now glutens (present in grains) are the biggest known triggers for autoimmune Hashimoto's disease (an autoimmune disorder that affects the thyroid gland). I find it interesting that the first recorded occurrences of thyroid issues in China coincided with the introduction of grains into their society.

In order to reap the benefits of a paleo/primal lifestyle, it is necessary to transition your body from a glucose-dependent sugar-burner to a fat-adapted fat-burner. The only negative in this transition is that it takes about three to four weeks of mental willpower to succeed. You don't have to lift a finger in terms of exercise in order to make this transition, but it does require a level of willpower as your body becomes un-addicted to glucose to fuel itself. During this period of transition, your brain will trick you into thinking you are hungry, and mental/physical energy lapses can occur. In actuality, your brain is an addict that is going through glucose/carbohydrate withdrawal and is trying to trick you into consuming its drug of choice—sugar.

Becoming fat adapted is the process of breaking an addiction cycle. One month of mental willpower for a lifetime of freedom was worth it to me. Becoming fat adapted not only changed my body, brain, and spirit, it enabled me to reduce my thyroid medication. Adopting a paleo lifestyle inherently addresses all of the underlying causes of adrenal fatigue and blood sugar issues which helps your endocrine system function more efficiently, including thyroid hormone metabolism.

Keys to Paleo Fat Adaptation
- Consume quality paleo/primal foods and manage carbohydrates (under 150 grams of total carbohydrates per day unless you are a professional athlete. For women or smaller people like me, under 100 grams of total carbohydrates per day or lower).
- Low-intensity exercise combined with an occasional sprint session.
- Lifestyle: getting adequate sleep, sunlight, fresh air, and stress reduction/management.
- General paleo/primal ratio: high fat/moderate protein/low carbohydrate.

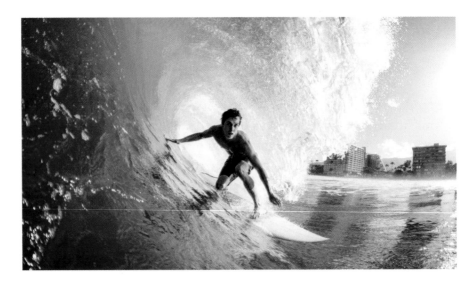

All four components of paleo/primal living must be adopted in order to achieve success in all areas, including weight loss, adrenal health, and blood glucose management.

We're going to explore the details of the paleo lifestyle, soon and I'll explain the principles listed at the beginning of this chapter, but first, some insight from the godfather of the paleo/primal/fat-burning world about why we all—even those not (yet!) experiencing thyroid problems—need to make an imperative change.

The Primal Blueprint

Mark Sisson, author of *The Primal Blueprint*, inspired me to go primal and become fat adapted, which was the final solution to the missing piece of the puzzle of my thyroid journey. I think his explanation behind the paleo principle of adopting a low-carbohydrate eating strategy is worth sharing.

INSULIN, BLOOD SUGAR & TYPE 2 DIABETES
from Mark Sisson's blog, MarksDailyApple.com
We all know by now that type 2 diabetes is an epidemic…

When you eat food, the body digests the macronutrients: carbohydrates, proteins—actually many different amino acids—and fats. Anything it can't digest, like alcohol or fiber or toxins, either passes right on through or, if it makes it into the bloodstream, gets filtered by your liver. We measure these in terms of grams and calories, but your body operates in terms of fuel. If you eat more fuel than your body needs (which most people do) the body is forced to store this excess. This ability to store excess fuel was an evolutionary imperative in a world that was in a state of constant "feast or famine" 50,000 years ago. In terms of primal health and our DNA blueprint, humans became very efficient fuel storage specialists and were able to survive the rigors of a hostile environment and pass those very same genes down to you and me.

Bear in mind that every type of carbohydrate you eat is eventually converted to a simple form of sugar known as glucose, either directly in the gut or after a brief visit to the liver. The truth is, all the bread, pasta, cereal, rice, fruit, dessert, and sodas you eat and drink eventually wind up as glucose. While glucose is a fuel, it is actually quite toxic in excess amounts unless it is being burned inside your cells, so the body has evolved an elegant way of getting it out of the bloodstream quickly and storing it in those cells. It does this by having the liver and the muscles store some of the excess glucose as glycogen. That's the muscle fuel that hard anaerobic exercise requires. Specialized beta cells in your pancreas sense the abundance of glucose in the bloodstream after a meal and secrete insulin, a peptide hormone whose job it is to allow glucose (and fats and amino acids) to gain access to the interior of muscle and liver cells. But there's the catch: once those cells are full, as they are almost all the time with inactive people, the rest of the glucose is converted to fat. Saturated fat.

Insulin was one of the first hormones to evolve in living things. Virtually all animals secrete insulin as a means of storing excess nutrients. It makes perfect sense that in a world where food was often scarce or non-existent for long periods of time, our bodies would become so incredibly efficient. How ironic, though, that it's not fat that gets stored as fat—it's sugar. *And that's where insulin insensitivity and this whole type 2 diabetes issue get confusing for most people, including our very own government.*

If we go back 10,000 or more years, we find that our ancestors had very little access to sugar—or any carbohydrates for that matter. There was some fruit here and there, a few berries, roots and shoots, but most of their carbohydrate fuel was locked inside a very fibrous matrix. In fact, some paleo-anthropologists suggest that our ancestors consumed, on average, only about 80 grams of carbohydrate a day. Compare that to the 350–600 grams a day in the typical American diet today. The rest of their diet consisted of varying degrees of fat and protein. And as fibrous (and therefore complex) as those limited carbohydrate foods were, their effect on raising insulin was minimal. In fact, there was so little carbohydrate/glucose in our ancestor's diet that we evolved four ways of making extra glucose ourselves and only one way of getting rid of the excess we consume.

Today when we eat too many carbohydrates, the pancreas pumps out insulin exactly as the DNA blueprint tells it to, but if the liver and muscle cells are already filled with glycogen, those cells start to become resistant to the call of insulin. The insulin "receptor sites" on the surface of those cells start to decrease in number as well as in efficiency. The term is called "down regulation." Since the glucose can't get into the muscle or liver cells, it remains in the bloodstream. Now the pancreas senses there's still too much toxic glucose in the blood, so it frantically pumps out even more insulin, which causes the insulin receptors on the surface of those cells to become even more resistant, because excess insulin is also toxic! Eventually, the insulin helps the glucose find its way into your fat cells, where it is stored as fat. Again—because it bears repeating—it's not fat that gets stored in your fat cells—it's sugar.

Over time, as we continue to eat high-carbohydrate diets and exercise less, the degree of *insulin insensitivity* increases. Unless we take dramatic steps to reduce carbohydrate intake and increase exercise, we develop several problems that only get worse over time—and the drugs don't fix it.

Ready for this? Let's go:

1. The levels of blood glucose stay higher longer because the glucose can't make it into the muscle cells. This toxic glucose is like sludge in the bloodstream clogging arteries, binding with proteins to form harmful AGEs (advanced glycated end-products) and causing systemic inflammation. Some of this excess glucose contributes to a rise in triglycerides, increasing risk for heart disease.

2. More sugar gets stored as fat. Since the muscle cells are getting less glycogen (because they are resistant), and since insulin inhibits the fat-burning enzyme lipase, now you can't even burn stored fat as easily. You continue to get fatter until eventually those fat cells become resistant themselves.

3. It just gets better. Levels of insulin stay higher longer because the pancreas thinks "if a little is not working, more would be better."

Wrong. Insulin is itself very toxic at high levels, causing, among many other maladies, plaque buildup in the arteries (which is why diabetics have so much heart disease) and increasing cellular proliferation in cancers.

4. Just as insulin resistance prevents sugar from entering muscle cells, it also prevents amino acids from entering. So now you can't build or maintain your muscles. To make matters worse, other parts of your body think there's not enough stored sugar in the cells, so they send signals to start to cannibalize your precious muscle tissue to make more—you guessed it—sugar. You get fatter and you lose muscle.

5. Your energy level drops, which makes you hungry for more carbohydrates and less willing to exercise. You actually crave more of the poison that is killing you.

6. When your liver becomes insulin resistant, it can't convert thyroid hormone T4 into the T3, so you get those mysterious and stubborn "thyroid problems," which further slow your metabolism.

7. You can develop neuropathies (nerve damage) and pain in the extremities, as the damage from the excess sugar destroys nerve tissue, and you can develop retinopathy and begin to lose your eyesight. Fun.

8. Eventually, the pancreas is so darn exhausted, it can't produce any more insulin and you wind up having to inject insulin to stay alive. Lots of it, since you are resistant and have insulin-dependent type 2 diabetes.

That's the bad news. And it's seriously bad. But the good news is that there is a way to avoid all this. It's all right there in your DNA blueprint. First off, exercise does have a major impact on improving insulin sensitivity since muscles burn your stored glycogen as fuel during and after your workout. Muscles that have been exercised desperately want that glucose inside and will "up regulate" insulin receptors to speed the process. That's one reason exercise is so critical for type 2 diabetics in regaining insulin sensitivity. It's also the reason why endurance athletes can eat 400 or 600 grams of carbohydrates a day and stay lean—they burn it all off and make room for more.

Resistance training seems to be as effective as aerobic activity, but a mix of the two is the best. And because you are now "insulin sensitive," you don't require as much insulin to store the excess, which "up regulates" all the fat-burning enzymes, so you burn your stored fats at a much higher rate throughout the day. Important amino acids and other vital nutrients have access to the cells when insulin sensitivity is high, so you're building or maintaining muscle and losing fat weight. Go team.

Second, cutting back on the carbohydrates, especially the obvious sugars and refined stuff is absolutely essential. While fresh vegetables should take up the bulk of space on your plate (that's still not many calories), the bulk of your calories should come from nutritious fat sources like high-quality meat, fish, fowl, and eggs, and high-fat plants like avocados, coconut, olives, nuts, and seeds. I get rip-roaring furious when I see our government suggesting that we get 60% of our calories from carbohydrates, grains in particular. That's ridiculous, bordering on criminal. Think about what is optimal for human health from a "primal" perspective. Look at the genetic blueprint. Look at the statistics and studies if you like—or simply observe what's going on around you at restaurants, movie theaters and school cafeterias—and you'll begin to understand the implications of a diet out of whack with our design. The evidence is nothing short of overwhelming: carbohydrate intake of the refined, sugary sort is enormously stressful to the body.

Not only should diabetics limit carbohydrate intake—everyone should.

We are all, in an evolutionary sense, predisposed to becoming diabetic.

Mainstream opinion is, of course, partly correct in that sugar does not necessarily "cause" diabetes—increasingly, scientific evidence is showing that genetic susceptibility plays a huge

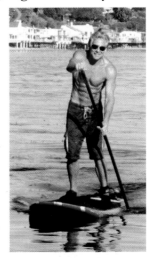

Mark Sisson on his paddleboard

role in individuals' potential for developing diabetes. Well, no kidding! The entire mainstream argument boils down to this: sugar does not cause diabetes; it's genetic. I couldn't agree more. I would simply say that our shared genetic susceptibility to insulin resistance, inflammation, cardiovascular disease, and obesity shows that any sort of refined sugar or grain is the last thing humans should be eating. Our genetic "primal blueprint" indicates that we are not meant to consume sugar.

For more information on Mark Sisson and *The Primal Blueprint*, visit MarksDailyApple.com and PrimalBlueprint.com.

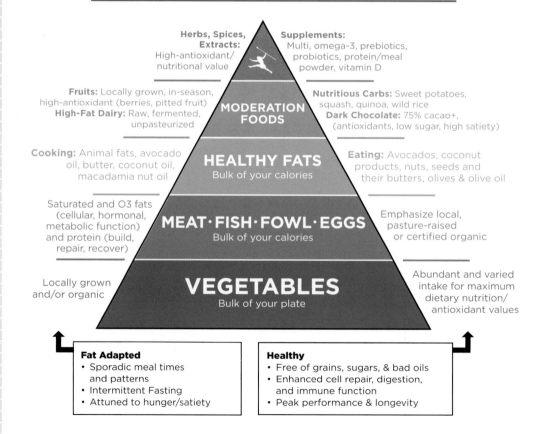

THE PRIMAL BLUEPRINT FOOD PYRAMID
Nutritious, satisfying, high nutrient value, low insulin stimulating foods.
Flexible choices and meal habits by personal preference.

Herbs, Spices, Extracts: High-antioxidant/ nutritional value

Supplements: Multi, omega-3, prebiotics, probiotics, protein/meal powder, vitamin D

Fruits: Locally grown, in-season, high-antioxidant (berries, pitted fruit)
High-Fat Dairy: Raw, fermented, unpasteurized

MODERATION FOODS

Nutritious Carbs: Sweet potatoes, squash, quinoa, wild rice
Dark Chocolate: 75% cacao+, (antioxidants, low sugar, high satiety)

Cooking: Animal fats, avocado oil, butter, coconut oil, macadamia nut oil

HEALTHY FATS
Bulk of your calories

Eating: Avocados, coconut products, nuts, seeds and their butters, olives & olive oil

Saturated and O3 fats (cellular, hormonal, metabolic function) and protein (build, repair, recover)

MEAT·FISH·FOWL·EGGS
Bulk of your calories

Emphasize local, pasture-raised or certified organic

Locally grown and/or organic

VEGETABLES
Bulk of your plate

Abundant and varied intake for maximum dietary nutrition/ antioxidant values

Fat Adapted
• Sporadic meal times and patterns
• Intermittent Fasting
• Attuned to hunger/satiety

Healthy
• Free of grains, sugars, & bad oils
• Enhanced cell repair, digestion, and immune function
• Peak performance & longevity

Getting Started with Paleo/Primal Living: Food First

"We are so off base from what we are genetically programmed to eat."
— Loren Cordain, author of *The Paleo Diet*

PALEO/PRIMAL FOOD LIST: FOOD FOR HUMANS!

Vegetables

Artichoke	Endive	Peppers (all kinds)
Arugula	Fennel	Pumpkin
Asparagus	Fiddlehead ferns	Purslane
Avocado	Garlic	Radish
Beets/beet greens	Green beans	Romaine lettuce
Bell peppers	Jerusalem artichoke	Rutabaga
Bok choy	Jicama	Sea vegetables
Broccoli	Kale	Spinach
Broccoli rabe	Kohlrabi	Swiss chard
Brussels sprouts	Leeks	Tomatoes
Cabbage	Mushrooms	Turnip greens
Carrots	Mustard greens	Watercress
Collards	Olives	
Cucumbers	Onions	
Eggplant	Parsnips	

Vegetables in Moderation

Cassava	Sweet potatoes	Wild rice
Potatoes	Taro	Yams

Fish

Anchovies	Mackerel	Rockfish
Bass	Mahimahi	Salmon
Catfish	Monkfish	Sardines
Cod	Mullet	Tilapia
Eel	Northern pike	Tuna
Haddock	Orange roughy	Walleye
Halibut	Perch	Any other wild fish
Herring	Red snapper	

Shellfish

Abalone	Lobster	Scallops
Clams	Mussels	Shrimp
Crab	Oysters	
Crayfish	Prawns	

Meat and Poultry

Beef	Goat	Pork
Chicken	Lamb	

Game Meat

Alligator	Emu	Rabbit
Bear	Goose	Snake
Buffalo	Pheasant	Turkey
Caribou	Kangaroo	Venison
Duck	Ostrich	
Elk	Quail	

Organ Meat

Bone Marrow	Kidney	Sweetbreads
Hearts	Liver	Tongue

Eggs

Chicken	Goose	Roe/Caviar
Duck	Pheasant	Other bird eggs
Emu	Quail	

Nuts and Seeds

Almonds	Macadamia	Pumpkin seeds
Brazil nuts	Pecans	Sesame seeds
Derivative butters	Pine nuts	Sunflower seeds
Hazelnuts	Pistachios	Walnuts

Healthy Fats/Oils

Avocado oil	Macadamia oil	Unprocessed palm oil
Butter/ghee	Olive oil	Walnut oil
Coconut oil/milk	Sesame oil	
Lard	Tallow	

Preferred Fruit

Blackberries	Boysenberries	Gooseberries
Blueberries	Cranberries	Raspberries

Other Fruits

Apple	Kiwi	Pineapple
Apricot	Lemon	Plums
Banana	Lime	Pomegranate
Cantaloupe	Lychee	Rhubarb
Cherries	Mango	Star fruit
Coconut	Nectarine	Strawberries
Fig	Orange	Tangerine
Goji berries	Papaya	Watermelon
Grapefruit	Passion Fruit	(And all others)
Grapes	Peach	
Guava	Pear	
Honeydew melon	Persimmon	

Spices and Herbs

Anise	Cumin	Parsley
Basil	Dill	Peppermint
Black pepper	Fennel	Rosemary
Cayenne pepper	Ginger	Sage
Chili pepper	Mint	Tarragon
Cilantro	Mustard seed	Thyme
Coriander seed	Nutmeg	Turmeric
Cinnamon	Oregano	
Cloves	Paprika	

Other

Beef gelatin protein powder	Probiotic
Bone broth	Stevia
Daily high-potency antioxidant multivitamin supplement	Tamari
	Tea (black, green, oolong, white
Fermented vegetables	Vinegar
Omega-3 fatty acid fish oil supplement	Vitamin D
	Whey Protein Powder

Dairy in Moderation

Cheese
Coffee
Full-fat cream
Yogurt

Occasional Indulgences

Alcohol
Dark chocolate

That list of food? It spells freedom. Going primal and becoming fat adapted will not only foster insulin sensitivity and thyroid hormone metabolism, but also it will banish food addictions. If you feel as if something is wrong with you because you are always thinking about food and what you are going to eat for your next meal, and/or you feel as though you use all of your willpower to prevent making bad food choices or overeating—it's not actually your fault! The sugar-burning state that your body is in (which promotes such food obsessions) was caused unintentionally. Likely, you were following conventional diet wisdom and didn't know any better, just like me.

So, how does one transition from being a sugar-burner to a fat-burner? There are many steps, but it starts with maintaining a level of carbohydrate intake below 150 total carbohydrates per day (and adjust from there to your own carbohydrate tolerance/threshold). The reason that a high-fat, moderate-protein diet is not dangerous when fat adapted is that the body doesn't have to worry about processing all the carbohydrates (excess glucose), so your body can instead focus on burning the fat on your body and the fat that you eat—for fuel. If you eat a high-fat, moderate-protein diet along with eating high carbohydrates, it's a recipe for disaster, because your body will be so busy trying to process the overload of sugar and deal with insulin levels that it won't have the "time" to properly process the fat and protein. All that unburned fat can cause cholesterol issues.

Mainstream thinking used to be that saturated fat was generally bad for you and caused heart disease. But we now know that saturated fat is not the culprit; eating a diet high in carbohydrates is. Saturated fat is essential to every cell in our body and is not a contributor to heart disease *unless* it's consumed in the presence of a chronically high-carbohydrate diet.

Let's explore the foods that are going to lead you away from those harmful carbs.

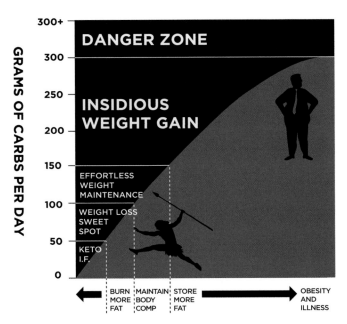

REMEMBER YOUR FAT/PROTEIN/CARBOHYDRATE LEVELS

This is very individual and you will intuitively discover what works for you after you have become fat adapted and have maintained a paleo lifestyle for four to six-plus weeks. While 120–150 carbohydrates a day might be appropriate for a large-framed man who is very physically active, 150 carbohydrates a day (the maximum level for a primal life-style) might be too much for your body. If you are sedentary, then 150 carbohydrates a day might be too much, but it is certainly better than anything *over* 150 carbohydrates a day, which is danger-zone territory. After much experimentation, I personally cannot tolerate 150 carbohydrates per day without experiencing weight gain. I have discovered that for my body, staying under 60–70 carbohydrates per day is best, and under 50 carbohydrates a day is even more ideal for me.

Do your best while becoming fat adapted and healing your body. The most important part of the process is becoming fat adapted, eliminating all the toxic food and oils in your diet, and adhering to eating food aligned with our your genetics. Master the paleo/primal food list *first* before worrying about which carbohydrate level under 150 per day is right for you and your body.

While a paleo/primal lifestyle usually means eating within a ratio of high-fat/moderate-protein/low-carbohydrate...this doesn't give you a license to eat all the fat or protein you want. You can gain body fat by eating more fat than you burn, and excess protein can turn into glucose. Experiment to find what levels of macronutrients are right for your body. What works for a 6'2" tall, muscular man would probably fail for a 5'2" short, petite woman. People with insulin resistance or a lot of excess body fat might need to drop their carbs low enough to ignite a state of ketosis in order to burn fat. Personal experimentation over time leads to an intuitive sense about what your body needs. 80% of body composition is determined by diet. Notice in the following example that the paleo graph in the center is a mirror opposite of the conventional one, except the carbs are replaced with fat. While this pattern offers a baseline from where to start, you are the only one who can dial it in and experience what works best for you.

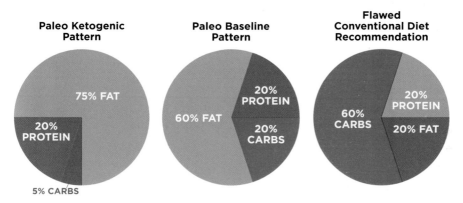

VEGETABLES AND FRUITS
Plants, both vegetables and fruits, form the basis of a paleo lifestyle even though they don't furnish the bulk of calories by any means. Vegetables and fruits provide volume, fiber, and other essential micronutrients. It's important that you eat the most nutritious, less problematic types. If you are trying to resolve insulin resistance and/or beat a sugar addiction, then vegetables can be viewed as your allies and fruits can be seen as your temporary enemies until insulin sensitivity returns and the sugar cravings disappear.

Growing Methods, in Order of Healthfulness

1. **Local organic:** The cream of the crop. Food from your neck of the woods, grown with organic methods. Eat food that doesn't have to travel halfway across the country to reach you.

2. **Local conventional:** Less transit time means a more recent harvest date, which means more nutrition. Local ranks higher than anything grown remotely, even organic. Remember that many smaller producers like the ones you'll run into at farmer's markets use organic methods without the official stamp of approval from the government. Cultivate a relationship with your farmers if you can. Many farmers are open to visitors coming and checking out their growing procedures, or helping with specific tasks like the labor-intensive potato harvest.

3. **Organic remote:** Produce grown without massive amounts of pesticides and herbicides applied tend to have higher levels of polyphenols, the plant's natural methods of protecting against pests and other aggressors. Those same polyphenols are good for us, too. If you have to eat food that's not local, go with this.

4. **Conventional remote with skin that's inedible or easy to wash:** If you're going to eat conventional produce, try to stick to vegetables whose skins you peel, remove, or easily wash. Avocados, onions, asparagus—these are pretty safe, since you're either not going to be eating the skin that's come into contact with chem-

icals or you'll be able to wash the skin effectively. For fruits, bananas, oranges, mangoes, pineapples, and kiwis are good.

5. **Conventional remote with edible or hard-to-wash surfaces:** Leafy greens, broccoli, bell peppers, and other vegetables whose surface area is eaten or too large to effectively wash should be eaten with caution or avoided altogether. Conventionally remotely grown fruits with soft, edible skin, like apples, apricots, peaches, plums, pears, grapes, berries, and tomatoes are best avoided.

Vegetable Nutritional Value

- **Nutrient dense:** *Beets, bell peppers, broccoli, Brussels sprouts, carrots, cauliflower, chard, eggplant, garlic, ginger, jicama, kale, onion, peas, romaine, spinach, and yellow squash are some of the vegetables with the highest levels of antioxidants, vitamins, minerals, and other beneficial components (like soluble fiber). Base your meals and your shopping around these vegetables and others from the list on page 117. Choose "heavy" vegetables, which in my entirely unscientific estimation, are more nutritious.*

- **Less nutrient dense:** *There's nothing wrong with vegetables like butter lettuce, cucumbers, or iceberg lettuce, but I wouldn't spend a lot of money on them when there are so many more intriguing and beneficial options available.*

Fruit Nutritional Value

- **Good antioxidant levels, low sugar:** *All berries, apricots, cherries, peaches, prunes.*
- **Good antioxidant levels, moderate sugar:** *Apples, bananas, figs, grapefruit, kiwi, pears, pomegranates.*
- **Good antioxidant levels, high sugar:** *Grapes, mangoes, melons, nectarines, oranges, papayas, pineapple, plums, tangerines.*

FISH, FLESH, AND EGGS

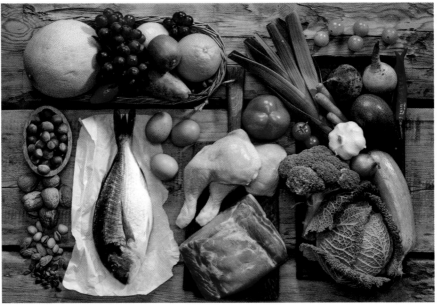

"Around 2 million years ago our ancestors were becoming more and more meat eaters and we feel that this had a great deal to do with expansion of the brain. Our bodies evolved (into) the way they are now, quickly….our brain however, took awhile to catch up. The high protein diet that they adopted developed our brains…we believe that it made all the difference in our evolution. If we had stayed as vegetarians, in all probability I wouldn't be speaking to you on this particular high level of intellect."

—Gary J. Sawyer, Physical Anthropologist, American Museum of Natural History (excerpt from the documentary *The Perfect Human Diet*)

Consuming fatty meat and complete protein from animal products supported the development of a complex brain that enabled us to ascend to the top of the food chain. But it's not just any meat that you should eat—just like fruits and vegetables, there's a hierarchy of healthfulness when it comes to meat and fish.

Paleo/primal living means doing your best to eat animals that are not fed grains—grains throw off the animal's fatty acid profile, which, in turn, can throw off yours. Also, animals fed in line with their DNA map tend to be more humanely raised, which is better for all of us. You wouldn't feed a horse a steak, because the DNA map for a horse dictates a different diet—a vegetarian one. An appropriate DNA-aligned diet for a cow does not involve grains. Ever wonder why some animals versus others are fed antibiotics? Well, when you feed cows grains (which is not aligned with their DNA map), they get sick. And when they get sick, they are administered antibiotics. I don't know about you, but I'll pass!

A popular misconception of paleo/primal living is that devotees, due to animal consumption, are contributing to the inhumane treatment of animals. But paleo living means adhering to how our hunter-gatherer ancestors ate, and our ancestors didn't feed animals grains or cram chickens together in small enclosures or farm fish; our ancestors only ate animals and fish that were living in the way nature intended them to live: roaming free and following their DNA-inspired diets.

Vegans and Vegetarians: Can They Be Paleo?

Archaeologically, we have measured thousands and thousands of human samples from all over the world, and we have yet to find a human that is a vegan or a vegetarian. In fact, when we start looking at humans from big villages where people were crowded together and consumed a high amount of grains in their diet, then you really see a difference in their bones. And these diseases that you would never see, you never saw in the Paleolithic, you start to see in kind of high abundances.—Mike Richards, Head of Archaeological Science Group, Department of Human Evolution at the Max Planck Institute for Evolutionary Anthropology (excerpt from the documentary The Perfect Human Diet*)*

While it would be virtually impossible (and also against our DNA blueprint) to attempt a paleo version of going vegan, vegetarians who consume *eggs (or pescatarians who eat fish) don't need to eat red meat in order to access all the benefits of fat adaptation and the paleo lifestyle. That said, if you are a vegetarian who consumes dairy products on a regular basis, limit your dairy intake to occasional while increasing your protein intake to **daily**.*

*My friend Eli Rohde (also a Primal Blueprint Certified Expert and primal coach), was a vegetarian for more than twenty years and experienced chronic arthritic inflammation until she discovered that grains and legumes were the culprits. After eliminating grains, legumes, and dairy from her life, the arthritic pain disappeared, but she was still hungry and tired often. For her, detaching from the identity as a hard-core vegetarian (and a proselytizing one) was difficult, but she took the leap and experimented for the sake of her health. Adopting a paleo/primal lifestyle completely transformed her life, and Eli is very devoted to the ancestral health movement and helping others achieve the same success she did. Eli now eats a myriad of primal foods, including marrow bones and organ meats! She regularly makes bone broth, brews her own kombucha, and ferments her own vegetables. The only time Eli experiences inflammation issues is when she consumes grains, which is either by accident or due to an **extremely rare** splurge (such as enjoying a croque monsieur on the streets of Paris). For Eli, quinoa causes the same inflammatory reactions in her body as grains do, so she stays away from pseudo-grains like quinoa as well.*

*If you are a vegan or a vegetarian who abstains from animal products based on ethical/moral grounds, I highly recommend reading **The Mindful Carnivore: A Vegetarian's Hunt for Sustenance** by Tovar Cerulli (or listen to my interview with him for free on **The Primal Blueprint** podcast).*

Animals were designed to roam pastured land and eat grass, insects, and so on. Consuming eggs from pasture-raised chickens or beef from 100% grass-fed or pasture-raised, cows or wild-caught fish is not only healthier, it contributes to sustainability. We can't always acquire grass-fed animal products (or organic produce or wild-caught fish) when dining out or traveling, so do your best at home to nourish yourself with the highest quality food.

THE PALEO THYROID SOLUTION

I visited a 100% grass-fed meat company that adopted the humane slaughtering techniques developed by a woman who revolutionized the cattle industry in the United States: Temple Grandin designed a system by which an animal could be led to its death in a calm, relaxed manner, unaware of its demise, even until the bullet enters its brain. When animals are stressed and aware that they are being led to slaughter, their cortisol levels rise significantly (as they would in humans faced with the same demise!). I don't know about you, but I would rather eat a healthy animal that lived and ate the way their DNA map intended, versus a grain-fed animal (which is a sick animal), that was also stressed to the max before slaughter.

Red Meat (Beef, Lamb, Pork), in Order of Healthfulness

1. **Grass-fed/grass-finished/pastured (pork):** Before organic and before local comes grass-fed and finished. Even a few weeks of grain feeding can alter the nutritional content and fatty acid composition of the resultant meat, so grass-fed and finished is the absolute best. These needn't be certified organic, but I've found that many grass-finished ranchers are organic in everything but name. You won't find grass-fed pork, because pigs aren't ruminants, but you can find pastured pork from pigs that are allowed to forage and often receive farm waste (milk, whey, fruits, vegetables).

   Note that "pastured" beef isn't necessarily grass-fed and finished. Bones, organ meat, and tougher cuts like chuck and stew are less expensive—and arguably more nutritious—ways to incorporate truly grass-finished animals into your diet. Many grass-fed/pastured meat companies can ship frozen animal products directly to your door, saving you the time and hassle of finding them locally. Red meat, along with seafood (and derivative fats), will likely provide the lion's share of your calories. Get the best possible product.

2. **Organic:** According to the United States Department of Agriculture (USDA), organic beef must come from cows must be

born and raised on organic pasture, must never receive antibiotics, must never receive growth-promoting hormones, must have unrestricted outdoor access, and must be fed only organic grasses and grains. So, yeah, grains. Note that there's no mention of the breakdown between grains and grasses; it could be 80% grains and 20% grass and still qualify as organic. So, while organic is clearly preferable to conventional meat, it's unlikely to be superior to grass-fed and finished meat without the organic label.

3. **CAFO:** Most meat you'll come across in supermarkets and restaurants will be from Concentrated Animal Feeding Operations (CAFO), where animals are treated like mere products and maximum productivity is prized above all else—even if it means pumping the animals full of antibiotics, hormones, and pesticide-laden feed. The resultant meat doesn't taste as good, it's less nutritious, and, at least in the case of pork, it's extremely high in omega-6 fats. In CAFOs animals are crammed together by the thousands or tens of thousands, often unable to breathe fresh air, walk outside, see the light of day, graze on plants or insects, or scratch the earth. A CAFO might slaughter and process a thousand cows per hour (a grass-fed/pasture-raised slaughterhouse of grass-fed/pasture-raised cattle might process ten cows per hour, and often the animals are *processed by hand*). Animals store toxins in their fat, so if you cannot order a grass-fed steak while out at a restaurant, then do your best to cut the fat off that steak and replace the fat by slathering on some delicious butter instead.

Poultry (and Eggs) in Order of Healthfulness

1. **Pastured:** A pastured chicken isn't just free range, given a patch of dirt upon which to scratch and peck; a pastured chicken is given access to pasture, to grassland teeming with a smorgasbord of delicious insects, nutritious plants, and edible seeds. The best pastured poultry gets most of its calories from the pasture, with a few handfuls of chicken feed to round things out back at the henhouse. Since poultry (and every animal we eat) doesn't create

nutrients out of thin air, its nutritional content is determined by the nutritional content of its diet. A pastured chicken (or duck, or turkey, or any farmed bird) tastes like a different animal altogether, probably because it's living like its primary ancestor—the jungle fowl—and its fatty acid composition bears that out (far less omega-6 than battery-raised birds). Same goes for eggs from said birds.

2. **Organic:** Organic poultry gets outdoor access and organic feed. It receives no antibiotics, no drugs, and no hormones (although that's true for all chickens, at least in the United States). It does not get access to pasture, to bugs, or to edible grasses unless otherwise specified. It's better than conventional poultry, but these birds are eating corn and soy (albeit non-GMO, organic) just the same.

3. **Free range:** Doesn't mean very much. The birds have access to the outside, but it's no more than a dirt patch. All the food (which is just soy and corn, of course) is inside, so that's where the birds will spend most of their time. At least these birds get to walk around some, rather than being crammed in a cage.

4. **CAFO:** Avoid if you can, unless you like eating beakless, stationary, big-breasted birds with soybean and corn oil for fat.

Seafood in Order of Healthfulness

The omega-3 fats, sea minerals like iodine, and other micronutrients seafood provides are essential—don't forget the iodine-depleted "Goiter Belt!" Even if you think you "hate" seafood, check out the lists below. I'm sure you'll be able to find something you can enjoy.

1. **Shellfish, farmed/wild; oily fish, wild; coho, farmed; barramundi:** Wild-caught sardines, salmon, tuna, anchovies, mackerel, and herring have the highest levels of omega-3 and, except for salmon and tuna, they're some of the most affordable fish around. Farmed shellfish are raised essentially like wild shellfish, attached to a fixed object and allowed to obtain sustenance from the ocean; they're also the most nutrient dense of the edible sea creatures.

And although most farmed salmon is nutritionally inferior to wild, farmed coho salmon is actually quite reminiscent of wild coho. Barramundi is fairly high in omega-3s, about the same as coho salmon. In the wild, it's omnivorous, but it does very well on a mostly herbivorous diet and needs far less fish meal than salmon while still retaining the omega-3s.

2. **Canned oily fish and shellfish:** Canned sardines, salmon, light tuna, oysters, mussels, and other fish from the first category are budget-friendly ways to eat healthy seafood. Just stick to BPA-free versions to avoid endocrine disruption.

3. **Domestic catfish, shellfish, trout, coho salmon, tilapia, barramundi, crayfish; non-oily wild fish:** While trying to farm wholly carnivorous fish is problematic and usually ends up producing an inferior food, replicating the diet of herbivorous fish is easier. In short, everything listed above is fair game, whether wild or farmed, especially if it's domestic. Neither they nor the non-oily wild fish like cod are particularly high in omega-3s, but they're all great sources of protein with decent levels of nutrients.

NUTS

Although all nuts are highly nutritious, they are calorically dense, and many of them are high in omega-6 fats. When you're talking about a whole food high in vitamin E and magnesium like an almond or a hazelnut, a little omega-6 isn't something to worry about. But when those occasional handfuls of nuts become regular, constant occurrences whose caloric content begins to approximate that of entire meals, the omega-6 fats add up.

Nuts in Order of Healthfulness

1. **Low omega-6 content** (indulge): Macadamia nuts reign supreme on this count.

2. **Moderate omega-6 content** (limit): Almonds, pistachios, cashews, hazelnuts.

3. **High omega-6 content** (avoid): Walnuts and pecans.

(Note that peanuts are *not* actually nuts, they promote inflammation, and they are often moldy. Not good!)

SUPPLEMENTAL CARBOHYDRATES

Most people can get all the carbohydrates they need from the "good" vegetables and the occasional bit of fruit. These supplemental carbohydrates should be used only to address a deficiency. If you're a hard-charging athlete who trains daily, then you might need some supplementary glucose to function best. If you're not, though, these foods should be eaten on a very *occasional* basis.

- **Tubers and other starchy vegetables:** Sweet potatoes of all kinds, potatoes of all kinds, and winter squash like butternut or acorn are all carbohydrate dense and nutrient dense, making them great sources of both supplemental carbohydrates for athletic purposes and of minerals, vitamins, and phytonutrients.

- **Wild rice, quinoa:** These pseudo-grains are gluten-free and relatively low in other plant toxins, especially if you soak and ferment them using traditional preparation methods. They're fine ways to add more glucose to your diet. However, some people experience the same adverse reactions that grains produce, and so be alert and aware of how they affect you.

DAIRY

If you are tolerant of dairy products, dairy can be a fantastic source of fat, protein, and nutrition. Stick to grass-fed and finished, or at least pastured, dairy products for the superior nutrition (CLA, vitamin K2).

Dairy products in Order of Healthfulness

1. **Raw, fermented, full-fat:** Think kefir and yogurt. Raw, fermented, full-fat dairy from a trusted, pastured supplier makes for the most nutritious, best-tasting, least-problematic choice. Fermentation takes care of most of the lactose, thus eliminating a potential agent of intolerance, while providing added probiotic benefits.

2. **Raw, full-fat:** Think butter, cream, whole milk. Raw dairy is more nutritious, its fats are less damaged, and the full-fat content is necessary for proper absorption and presence of fat-soluble vitamins like A and K2. Plus, full-fat dairy contains the most conjugated linoleic acid (CLA).

3. **Organic, non-homogenized, full-fat:** Sure, it's pasteurized, but at least the fat globules haven't been damaged after undergoing high-pressure homogenization. The fat-soluble vitamins will be mostly intact.

FAT: FABULOUS AND ESSENTIAL

Again, dietary fat is *good* for you. You *need* it. If you eat a lot of good fat as part of a paleo lifestyle, you will be *leaner, healthier,* and *more resilient.* Many people are hesitant to introduce fat to their diets, because they're worried about gaining weight or because they are trying to be "heart healthy." There is zero correlation between the consumption of foods high in saturated fat or high in cholesterol and the risk of heart disease.

Here is how heart disease manifests: excess consumption of carbohydrates (grains and sugars) promotes excess insulin production and high triglycerides in the bloodstream. Along with consumption of unhealthy oils and a stressful lifestyle (not enough sleep, not enough sun, chronic exercise), this pattern promotes a state of oxidation and inflammation in the bloodstream. Under these circumstances, cholesterol in the bloodstream can then turn dangerous, with small, dense LDL molecules becoming lodged on artery walls and sustaining oxidative damage. This elicits an immune system response that leads to further inflammation, the formation of plaque on the artery walls, and an eventual heart attack or stroke.

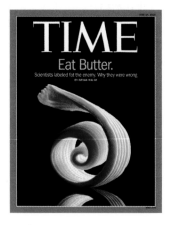

I jumped for joy when I saw this cover of *Time* magazine: a huge step toward ending the war on fat in our country and turning the tables on high-carbohydrate diets.

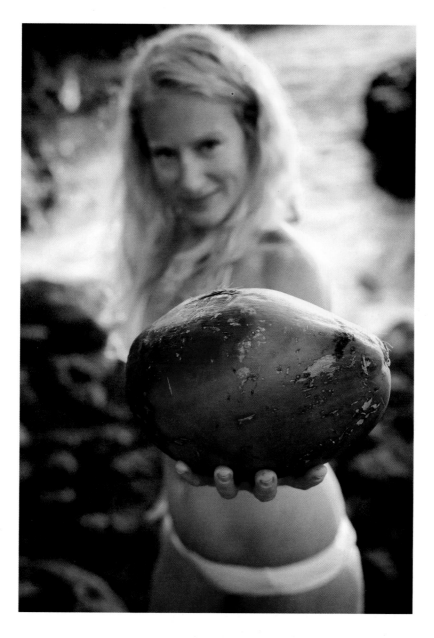

Coconuts are a great source of healthy fat.

Dietary Fats: Dietary fats come in different forms, offering an assortment of health benefits and, in some cases, compromising health. Dietary fats are commonly distinguished by whether they are solid at room temperature (known as "saturated") or liquid (known as "unsaturated"). Many fats contain a blend of different types of fat molecules. For example, olive oil is commonly characterized as a monounsaturated fat because it contains 78% monounsaturated fatty acids, but it is also comprised of 14% saturated fatty acids, and 8% polyunsaturated fatty acids.

Saturated: With saturated fats, all potential bonding sites on the carbon atoms of the fatty acid chain are occupied by hydrogen, hence the term "saturated." Saturated fat, often erroneously maligned by conventional wisdom as contributing to the heart disease process, is an excellent source of caloric energy with no known adverse health effects. Saturated fats contribute to critical metabolic functions, including enhanced nutrient absorption and immune function and protection against oxidative damage (our cell membranes are made of saturated fat). Only when saturated fats are consumed in the presence of excessive carbohydrates, such as with the Standard American Diet (SAD), can they be potentially troublesome. As Gary Taubes asserts in *Why We Get Fat*, there has never been a single scientific study showing that saturated fats, by themselves, are unhealthy.

Saturated fats are commonly found in animal foods (meat, eggs, butter, cream) or in certain tropical oils, such as coconut and palm. They are extremely temperature stable and thus resistant to oxidative damage when they are exposed to heat, light, or oxygen. This makes saturated fats such as butter, lard, and coconut oil preferred choices for cooking.

Monounsaturated: These fats contain a single double bond ("mono") in their fatty acid chain. Monounsaturated fats are universally regarded as healthy, lauded for enhancing cardiovascular and immune function and offering protection against heart disease.

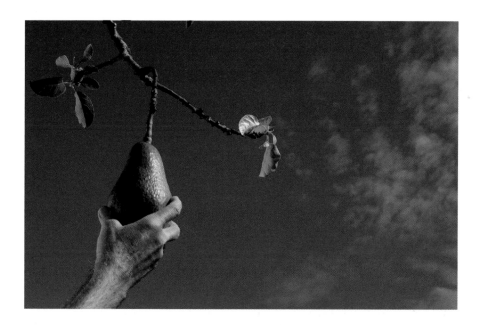

Good sources of monounsaturated fat include Macadamia nuts, avocado, olives, and extra-virgin olive oil. They are less temperature stable than saturated fats, and thus should not be used for high-temperature cooking. However, olive oil can tolerate mild warming temperatures without oxidizing.

The Standard American Diet (SAD), high in grains, vegetable and seed oils, and chemically altered fats, brings numerous health objections, particularly that these foods have minimal nutritional value and cause oxidative damage in the body.

Polyunsaturated: These fats contain more than one double bond in their fatty acid chain. The more double bonds a fatty acid contains, the more fluid it is. Hence, these oils retain their liquid form at room temperature and even when refrigerated. However, polyunsaturated fatty acids (PUFAs) are highly susceptible to damage from even routine exposure to light, heat, and oxygen, something that commonly occurs during the manufacturing process, not to mention when they are used for cooking!

The most common forms of PUFA in today's diet are vegetable seed oils, such as canola, corn, soy, safflower, and sunflower. Other high PUFA foods include butter-like spreads, salad dressings, and assorted packaged and processed snack foods made with these offensive oils. Cooking with a PUFA oil, like canola, produces significant oxidative damage to the molecules. The endocrine system is especially vulnerable to the ingestion of oxidized PUFA, which can lead to disruption in healthy hormone and immune function.

Omega-6 and Omega-3: Polyunsaturated fatty acids are divided into two categories of essential fatty acids ("essential" meaning fat we cannot manufacture internally and must obtain from our diet): omega-6 fatty acids and omega-3.

Omega-3 fatty acids: These fats are named for the hydrogen double bond at the third carbon in the fatty acid chain. Lauded for enhancing cardiovascular, brain, skin, and immune function, omega-3s help moderate systemic inflammation, increase insulin sensitivity, and reduce the risk of heart attack, arthritis, autoimmune disorders, and cognitive issues such as depression, ADHD, and Alzheimer's.

Omega-3s are found in highest concentration in oily, cold-water fish (herring, mackerel, wild salmon, sardines, tuna). Pasture-raised eggs and animal meats are also good sources of omega-3s, as are leafy greens. Nuts and seeds contain significant levels of omega-3s as well, but are invariably higher in omega-6 than omega-3.

Omega-6 fatty acids: These fats are named for the hydrogen double bond at the sixth carbon in the fatty acid chain. Omega-6 fats from nutritious foods offer assorted health benefits, but unfortunately the excess consumption of these fats (along with insufficient omega-3 intake) via unhealthy food sources is common.

Omega-6 fatty acids are found in healthy foods such as nuts and seeds, but also in vegetable oils, conventionally raised animals fed grain-based diets (at the expense of the animal's omega-3 levels, which might be more elevated if the animal was raised in the pasture, eating omega-3–containing grasses instead of grain feed high in omega-6), bakery items (doughnuts, cookies), and all manner of processed, packaged, and frozen foods.

The dietary ratio of omega-6 to omega-3 fatty acids has become a popular topic in evolutionary health circles. The main concern is insufficient intake of omega-3s, which are widely regarded as healthful and anti-inflammatory, coupled with an excess intake of omega-6s, which are widely regarded as pro-inflammatory.

Breaking research suggests that this may be an oversimplification of the issue, that in fact both omega-6 and omega-3 have anti-inflammatory properties. However, omega-3s have a stronger anti-inflammatory effect. What happens when we ingest linoleic acid–the primary omega-6 fatty acid–is that it converts into arachidonic acid (AA), generally a precursor for inflammatory cytokines and thus labeled as "pro-inflammatory." When we ingest alpha-linoleic acid (ALA), the plant form of omega-3 fatty acid, it converts into the anti-inflammatory precursors EPA and DHA (as seen on fish oil capsules). These conversions happen on the same enzymatic pathways, so they are competing for limited access to our cells. When we consume an excess of linoleic acid, our conversion of ALA into EPA and DHA is compromised, leading to a potential inflammatory imbalance. However, this imbalance can be countered with direct consumption of foods or supplements high in EPA and DHA, such as oily, cold-water fish, pasture-raised animals and eggs, or high-quality fish oil supplements.

The Standard American Diet (SAD), high in grains, vegetable and seed oils, and chemically altered fats, brings numerous health objections, particularly that these foods have minimal nutritional value and cause oxidative damage in the body. Industrial oils, processed grain-based snacks, and CAFO animals all happen to be high in omega-6, contributing to a high ratio of omega-6 to omega-3. Again, the ratio could be of secondary concern to the lack of sufficient omega-3 intake and the excessive intake of unhealthy foods that happen to be high in omega-6. For example, it's estimated that the SAD eater obtains around 70% of their (mostly omega-6) polyunsaturated fatty acids from industrial oils, shortening, and margarine. Only small percentages of total omega-6 intake come from nuts, seeds, beans, and animal products. Consequently, omega-6 fatty acids should not been seen as unhealthy per se, but rather that the elevated omega-6 to omega-3 ratio is a symptom of poor dietary habits, and that much of our omega-6 fatty acids come from rancid oils, fast-food products cooked in oil, and packaged snacks and treats made with shortening/partially hydrogenated oils, and other processed foods high in sugar and industrialized oils.

Both omega-6 and omega-3 fats are "essential" to consume to promote a healthy inflammatory balance, among other functions, in the body. It's also important to keep in mind that "inflammation" is not entirely bad either. The inflammatory process is a critical element of healthy immune function and the fight-or-flight response for peak performance. Brief bouts of inflammation triggered by high-intensity exercise helps build fitness and promotes optimal gene expression. Similarly, the inflammation that occurs at an injury site (sprained ankle, bee sting, black eye) allows the cellular damage to be contained in that one area instead of circulating throughout the bloodstream, and also speeds the healing process by increasing blood flow and accelerating the removal of waste products in that area.

It is only when inflammation is chronic or system-wide that health is compromised and risk is elevated for high blood pressure, coronary artery disease, depressed immune function, suboptimal neurological function, and many other health problems and serious diseases. Chronic or systemic inflammation is caused by poor dietary habits (too many processed foods, too little omega-3 intake), and high-stress lifestyle behaviors such as excessive exercise, insufficient sleep, and poor work/leisure balance.

Hunter-gatherer references: It's commonly mentioned that our hunter-gatherer ancestors had an omega-6:omega-3 ratio of 1:1, or at least

2:1. This was due to the absence of eating the aforementioned high omega-6 processed foods and the likelihood of obtaining higher levels of omega-3s from typical hunter-gatherer fare. Today, the typical SAD eater has an estimated ratio of 20:1 or even worse. While this gross imbalance in comparison to our hunter-gatherer ancestors presents a compelling sound bite, it's best to focus on the big-picture task of increasing omega-3 intake for the broad health benefits (especially the anti-inflammatory effects), along with eliminating unhealthy foods that happen to be high in omega-6 to protect yourself from oxidative damage.

Trans and Partially Hydrogenated Fats: These chemically altered fats are similar but not identical. Hydrogenation is a process by which an unsaturated fat (typically a vegetable oil) is heated to a high temperature under extreme pressure and mixed with toxic metallic solvents to saturate the carbon bonds with hydrogen and render the fat solid at room temperature. In food manufacturing, the typical method is to partially saturate the carbon bonds, rendering the fat solid (saturated) at room temperature but able to melt upon baking or consumption.

"Trans" refers to the presence of hydrogen on both sides of the carbon chain. Trans fats occur naturally in certain foods, such as cow's milk and meat, in trace amounts. In their natural form, they are known as conjugated linoleic acid (CLA) or vaccenic acid. The process of hydrogenation creates a trans fat of distorted shape, rendering the molecule straighter than its natural, slightly bent, composition. Since the process of hydrogenation alters fat molecules into the trans form (the normal shape is known as "cis" form), all partially hydrogenated fats are trans fats, but not vice versa. The creation of a trans fat can be considered an undesirable side effect of the partial hydrogenation process. To distinguish between the healthy, natural trans fats found in whole foods and the chemically altered partially hydrogenated trans fats discussed here, we will refer to the latter as "chemically altered trans fats" for the duration of this section.

Chemically altered trans fats are easily oxidized to form free radical chain reactions that damage cell membranes, promote systemic inflammation, obesity, immune system dysfunction, the oxidation and inflammation process that characterizes heart disease, and many other serious health problems. These chemically altered trans fats are unable to be metabolized normally by the body, but your body is fooled into incorporating these agents into fat-based cell membranes. Incorporating dysfunctional synthetic fat molecules into your cell membranes contributes directly to inflammation, aging, cancer, and heart disease. Medical experts estimate that as many as 100,000 premature deaths from cancer and heart disease annually can be directly attributed to the routine consumption of trans fats in the Western diet.

Chemically altered trans fats are found in the majority of conventionally processed, packaged, frozen, and fast-food products (for example, crackers, chips, cookies, pastries, doughnuts, shortening, and deep-fried fast foods). Consumer awareness about the extreme dangers of consuming chemically altered trans fats is growing, leading many food manufacturers and restaurants to avoid using these agents. For example, New York City has banned the use of trans fats in all restaurants since 2008.

A new category of fat called *interesterified fats* has been introduced into the marketplace to avoid the now-notorious trans fat labeling. These fats are also created through a type of hydrogenation process that alters their molecular structure and renders them problematic for ingestion.

PROBIOTICS FOR GUT HEALTH

Gut health is key to healthy thyroid hormone metabolism, health, and longevity. The state of the bacteria in the intestinal tract influences many elements of health. The immune system in particular depends upon a healthy balance of bacteria in the gastrointestinal tract, a state characterized by a predominance of "friendly" bacteria over the "bad" bacteria that can cause illness. Unless you are consuming fermented foods on a regular basis, supplementing with probiotics is essential for strong immunity and T4 to T3 thyroid hormone conversion. Our hunter-gatherer ancestors ingested dirt and soil with every meal, along with billions of beneficial microorganisms in the form of bacteria and yeast. To optimize our health, our genes developed a reliance on a regular and consistent supply of these soil-based organisms. So with every bit of dirt ingested, our ancestors were strengthening their immune and digestive systems—improving their health with every bite. So must we.

ELIMINATE GRAINS AND LEGUMES

"Here's the deal with 'whole grains.' Do grains contain some valuable nutrients? Sure. But so do tree bark, grass, twigs, and other foods that don't jibe with human physiology. It's not surprising that diets including whole grains result in better health outcomes than diets rich in *refined* grains, but that doesn't mean they are an optimal choice—whole grains are just the lesser of some other Neolithic evils. Whole grains block the absorption of a lot of the nutrients we need and can increase your appetite. **If we were comparing grain-based vs. grain-free diets, the truth of their effects would come to light, much to the chagrin of every company touting the benefits of whole grains…which is just a marketing gimmick anyway.**"

—Mark Sisson, author of *The Primal Blueprint*

This concept is hard for grain-lovers to digest, *literally*, because humans were not programmed to consume grains. So many people are not only addicted to grain-based foods, but also they've been told by the government and advertising campaigns that whole grains are healthy and are a big part of what keeps us healthy—not true. In fact, the opposite is true.

Grains include wheat, corn, rice, pasta, cereals, cooking grains (barley, millet, rye, oats, etc.), and all derivatives, such as bread, pasta, crackers, snack foods, cookies, cakes, candies, and assorted other types of processed, packaged, frozen, and fresh-baked goods.

Grains are just a cheap source of calories that are converted into glucose. Some people claim, "I don't have a sweet tooth." Well, if you eat grains you do! A piece of bread turns into glucose faster in the body than a spoonful of cane sugar!

Carbohydrates = Glucose/Sugar

Grains have minimal nutritional value, stimulate excess insulin production, and contain anti-nutrients that compromise digestive and immune function, promote systemic inflammation, and inhibit the absorption of vitamins and minerals.

- -

Can You Do It? Of *Course* You Can!

*It may seem daunting to give up grains, but be honest with yourself: have you ever truly enjoyed eating a grain **by itself**? I am betting the answer is no, because in order to make grains palatable, we usually add butter, sauce, sugar, fruit, or something else to it. Does anyone eat plain pasta **without butter**? A plain bagel **without** cream cheese? I would love to meet a person who claims to love the taste of "plain" grains, but I doubt that person exists. Think about it: **fat** is what makes grains tasty—the butter on toast, the butter and sauce on pasta, the cream cheese or nut butter on a bagel. However, grains completely fail on their own; without fat or sugar added to them, grains are nothing more than toxic, beige sludge that does humans a lot of harm and triggers the onset of autoimmune disorders like Hashimoto's.*

Besides, with the plethora of paleo cookbooks available and paleo websites offering hundreds of free paleo recipes...grain-free muffins, bread, pizza crusts, and pasta can still be a part of your paleo lifestyle. That said, I strongly

----

Grains and legumes *compromise* nutrition rather than encourage it.

Grains are the biggest known triggers of autoimmune disorders, particularly Hashimoto's. Any nutrients in grains are likely canceled out by the anti-nutrients they contain. People think brown rice is healthier than white rice—not so. Whole grains contain higher levels of anti-nutrients. Legumes have a higher nutritional value and fewer anti-nutrients than grains do, but legumes are unnecessary to consume because of their high-carbohydrate load and propensity to disturb digestion. Grains and legumes *compromise* nutrition rather than encourage it.

> "Grains cause a chronic inflammatory state of the gut and are a big initiator of almost all of our inflammatory diseases and autoimmune diseases. Rheumatoid arthritis was virtually absent from the archaeological record until the introduction of grains into the human diet."
> —Lane Sebring, MD
> (excerpt from the documentary *The Perfect Human Diet*)

ELIMINATE OR LIMIT ALCOHOL

I personally dislike alcohol because I can feel the effects of its toxicity in my body and brain. The day after I consume any amount of alcohol (even one glass), I become unfocused, lethargic, and depressed (after all, alcohol is a *depressant*). I understand that this is a sensitive topic for a lot of people who feel the need for a daily glass of wine or two. Of course, the best course of action would be to quit drinking alcohol entirely while you are trying to heal your thyroid and adrenals—I know that is easier said than done. If you cannot abstain from alcohol, muster the willpower to limit your intake to one glass a day instead of two or more, and then try to eventually limit the intake to a few days a week, versus every day.

Alcohol has a negative effect on body composition goals as a source of "empty calories" (7 calories per gram) and is a potential contributor to insulin resistance. Contrary to popular belief, alcohol does not convert into fat upon ingestion. Rather, alcohol is absorbed directly into the bloodstream and has an immediate effect on the brain and other tissues; hence, the resulting "buzz." Since alcohol is a toxin, the body works quickly to metabolize the alcohol through oxidation. This detoxifies and removes the alcohol from the bloodstream before it damages organs and tissues. In the liver, enzymes convert alcohol into acetaldehyde and then acetate. This is what happens to most of the alcohol consumed, but some alcohol escapes the metabolic process and is excreted unchanged through the breath or urine.

> *As the "first to burn" calorie source, alcohol inhibits fat metabolism, makes carbohydrates more likely to be converted into fat, and can stimulate increases in appetite.*

While alcohol is being burned or converted into acetate, metabolism of other fuels is put on hold. Hence, alcohol calories are known as the "first to burn." Not only is fat burning put on hold while the alcohol calories are burned, but *any carbohydrate calories consumed with alcohol are more likely to be converted into fat and stored instead of burned.* Similarly, fat calories consumed with alcohol will more likely be stored as fat instead of burned (if they were being consumed without insulin-stimulating carbohydrates).

Kansas City Public Library
Waldo Library
201 East 75th Street
Kansas City, MO 64114
816 701 3486

Customer ID: *********8072

Items that you checked out

Title: The paleo thyroid solution
ID: 0000183780709
Due: Monday, December 12, 2022
Messages:
Charged

Total items: 1
Account balance: $0.00
11/21/2022 5:44 PM
Checked out: 1
Overdue: 0
Hold requests: 0
Ready for pickup: 0

Thank you

Since alcohol inhibits lipolysis (fat burning) and glycolysis (glucose burning) being the first to burn, studies correlate frequent consumption with hypoglycemia (low blood sugar). In fact, according to Enoch Gordis, MD, director of the National Institute on Alcohol Abuse and Alcoholism (NIAAA), the stupor commonly associated with drunk people could often be more due to hypoglycemia than the effects of alcohol. A pattern of frequent alcohol consumption can also result in decreased insulin sensitivity and elevated levels of the key appetite-stimulating hormone ghrelin. The blood sugar imbalances caused by frequent alcohol consumption can negatively affect the adrenal glands, thereby stunting optimal hormone and thyroid hormone metabolism.

If you get the munchies in correlation with alcohol intake, it is validated by science! And when you do eat, those calories are more likely to be stored as fat. Alcohol ingestion thus detracts from fat loss goals by contributing empty calories (that you will burn before tapping into stored body fat), interfering with other ingested calories (promoting the conversion of ingested carbohydrates into fat), and increasing appetite. Along those lines, if alcohol is to be consumed, it is best consumed alone to mitigate fat storage concerns, and, of course, in a sensible and moderate manner.

Alcohol can also affect body composition by altering the healthy balance of sex hormones in both males and females. Alcohol is known to be directly toxic to the testes, lowering testosterone levels in males. Frequent consumption can disturb hormone functions in the hypothalamus and pituitary glands, damage sperm, and compromise fertility. In premenopausal females, frequent alcohol consumption can cause an assortment of reproductive problems, including abnormal menstrual cycles, delayed ovulation, and infertility. These negative effects are well associated with alcoholics, but reproductive issues can also occur in "social" drinkers.

In postmenopausal women, alcohol has been found to promote elevated levels of estradiol (estrogen), which commonly falls dramatically after menopause. The elevated blood estrogen levels from moderate alcohol consumption can actually deliver some health benefits by helping to reduce the risk of cardiovascular disease without increasing the risk of bone loss, liver disease, or breast cancer. Due to the toxic effects of alcohol and its negative influence the healthy metabolism of other calories, anything beyond occasional, casual drinking will have a negative effect on healthy metabolic and hormonal function.

Getting rid of alcohol in your life will not only assist in fat loss, but also its absence will ensure that your fat-adaptation won't get thrown out of whack by negatively affecting your blood sugar and insulin levels. Do your best to eliminate alcohol from your life while working toward resolving your thyroid issues. If you can't eliminate it, *dial back significantly*.

FASTING

It may seem counterintuitive, but fasting now and then (even from after bedtime to noon the following day) can be a valuable part of a paleo/primal lifestyle. It offers benefits like increased longevity, neuroprotection, increased insulin sensitivity, stronger resistance to stress, increased mental clarity, and more.

Just eat according to the primal principles I've laid out for you, and once you are fat adapted and have healthy adrenal function and optimal thyroid hormone levels, experiment with skipping meals occasionally. A sixteen-hour fast is on the low-but-still-effective end (you could easily do it daily, eating all your food within an eight-hour window), or you could opt for longer, more intermittent fasts—say, a full twenty-four hours once or twice a week. When you're done with the fast, eat as much as you want (overeating usually isn't an issue, once you're fat adapted).

This plan essentially turns into "eat when you're hungry," because let's face it: eating the types of foods we evolved eating induces powerful satiety and makes eating the right amount of food a subconscious act. Fasting becomes a whole lot easier (and more intuitive) when you've got your food quality dialed in.

If fasting scares you or you find that it doesn't quite align with your mental energy needs (or your supplement regimen), instead of 100%

fasting, you can try what I do: instead of eating a full meal during the hours after waking until noon or 1:00 p.m., I will eat a small amount of fat (like a tablespoon of coconut oil, or ½ to ¼ of an avocado with salt, or a very tiny amount of protein and fat together.) This not only continues to train the body to use fat as fuel, but it also helps when you have to take certain supplements with food in the first half of the day.

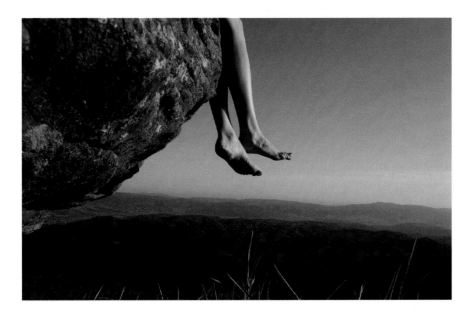

Just Because It's Well-Meaning
Doesn't Make It Less Wrong

I came across this thyroid book online.

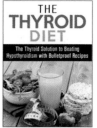

Now, I have not read The Thyroid Diet; for all I know, the author could be giving great health advice in her book. Regardless, the cover photo is alarming and sends a very misguided message and is a classic example of a flawed, conventional approach. Notice that the foods on the cover are all carbohydrates—the most concerning being the rice cakes and the large glass of orange juice. A glass of orange juice has 25 grams of carbohydrates and 20 grams of sugar. The six rice cakes in the photograph total 42 grams of carbohydrates. The orange juice and rice cakes together equal 67 grams of carbohydrates. (The salad and veggies have an extremely low carbohydrate count, so I won't bother factoring them in here.) Anyone who eats this meal is going to be hungry a few hours later and experience a drop in energy, because there is nothing satiating about these foods (and these foods contribute to blood sugar spikes, which will affect adrenals and inhibit fat loss). Fat and protein are technically the only two food categories that humans require for health, and they are nowhere to be found in this cover photo. For people trying to consume around 100 carbohydrates a day or lower (a carbohydrate level worthy of most people who are moderately physically active)—and considering that our ancestors likely consumed less than 80 grams of carbohydrates a day—

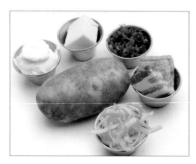

the grouping of foods on this book cover is a joke when it comes to carbohydrate management. I don't know about you, but I would rather have a "loaded" baked potato with bacon, chives, sour cream, and butter instead of six rice cakes and a glass of orange juice (1 large baked potato = 63 grams carbohydrates).

Paleo/Primal Exercise

Our hunter-gatherer ancestors not only did plenty of low-intensity walking and dynamic functional body movements, they didn't overdo it on exercise, and they had a lot of time to recover from physical activity. When a person engages in physical activity and exceeds 75% of their maximum heart rate for extended periods of time (chronic cardio), they are burning glucose. As a fat-burner, you don't want to do that because you will deplete your glucose stores and will need to replace them, which can ignite a sugar-burning cycle.

How does this relate in the real world? A lot of people engage in chronic cardio at glucose-burning high intensities. You want to stay between 55% and 75% of your maximum heart rate, except for random short bursts as in the case of a weekly sprint session or other weekly high-intensity workout. Here's a classic sugar-burning scenario: you have to eat every two or three hours or your blood glucose levels drop and fluctuate, so you become a slave to food. And because of your higher carbohydrate consumption you will need to burn the glucose in order to achieve a lean physique, which puts one on a never-ending hamster wheel of burning glucose and consuming glucose (carbohydrates).

Have you ever thought or heard someone say, "I just don't understand...I work out every day and eat right and I'm still not losing weight." That is what happens when one gets trapped in the sugar-burning cycle. Being a sugar-burner can lead to developing hypoglycemia. And if you have hypoglycemia, the way to *reverse* it is to become fat adapted, which will manage blood glucose levels and prevent hypoglycemic spikes that occur when someone is a slave to their fluctuating blood sugar levels. When blood glucose spikes and drops chronically, adrenal glands suffer and people experience unnecessary surges in cortisol. The body reads the highs and lows of glucose as a stress and sends cortisol to respond.

EXERCISE OPTIONS

I do something physically active for at least thirty to sixty minutes every day (and occasionally two to three hours).

Swimming: If I feel lazy, I go for a thirty-six-lap swim in a 25 yard pool, which takes me about twenty-two minutes and equals half a mile. Now, I know it sounds insane that I find swimming "lazy," but here's why: I swim with a snorkel and a mask. Have you ever been snorkeling? It's *fun*! Not only can I breathe deeply whenever I want, I can go faster and longer than swimmers who use goggles, because they have to continuously crank their necks to the side and gasp for short bursts of air (swimming in that way is stressful to me, negatively affects my neck and shoulders, and is not fun for me at all). Swimming with a snorkel and a mask, on the other hand, makes swimming fun, meditative, and even easier on the body because the floatation factor increases with a snorkel and mask, so the body becomes more aligned at the surface of the water. Swimming (or any pool exercise) is also a great one-stop-shop for full-body conditioning and can be the perfect exercise for people with injuries. In fifteen to twenty minutes, you can log a full-body workout and a stretch routine at the same time. I swim two to four days a week, depending. Chlorine is considered anti-thyroid, so if you are trying to fix a thyroid problem naturally, I suggest staying away from chlorinated pools and water altogether. Whenever possible, swim in fresh salt water or saline pools.

Hiking: There is nothing more enjoyable in my opinion, than being outside in nature and strolling up and down a mountain trail. I wear a heart rate monitor and make sure that I hike slow and steady and stay within 55%–75% of my maximum heart rate. Hiking is more enjoyable when approached with a slow and steady pace versus hauling ass up a mountain. And hiking at a slower pace ensures fat-burning versus sugar-burning. I live in the mountains where there are endless amounts of trails. I hike three to seven days a week for an hour, and once a week I do a two- to three-hour hike with a friend.

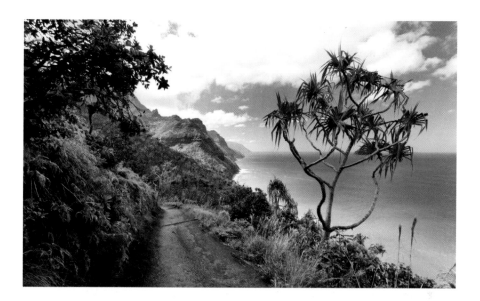

Walking: I love walking on the beach because it works different muscles than walking on concrete with shoes. But most of the time I just walk out my front door with a good audiobook or podcast cued up in my iPhone, and I walk around my neighborhood for thirty to forty-five minutes. If it's raining or cold outside and I decide to hit the treadmill at my gym, I usually bring my iPad and watch part of a film or a TV show while I walk for thirty to sixty minutes (usually at a slower pace, between 2.8 and 3.3 mph). I find being on a treadmill incredibly boring, but time really flies by whenever I watch something, or listen to music or a podcast. For those of you living in cold climates, you might want to try walking longer than expected if your attention is focused on something enjoyable versus staring at the treadmill dashboard, watching time creep by slowly. Of course you can apply this strategy to any cardio machine endeavor at the gym.

Pilates: I love Pilates, but it can be a very pricy exercise choice when doing classical "reformer Pilates." However, Pilates is still accessible to all for free: there are many "mat Pilates" videos available on YouTube and elsewhere. Pilates is wonderful for spinal alignment, full-body conditioning, core strength, and flexibility.

Sprinting: This high-intensity training is a great way to get results in a very short period of time, and it is hormonally beneficial when stress hormones are raised temporarily in this way (versus chronically), contributing to increased fat-burning and human growth hormone. Running all-out, as fast as you can, for fifteen to thirty seconds, catching your breath and then doing it again (repeating four to seven times) usually takes no more than ten to fifteen minutes! You get a lot of bang for your buck on this one. While high-intensity training on a chronic, daily basis can be detrimental, sprinting every seven to ten days is ideal for changing your body composition, and your DNA blueprint encourages it.

Lift Heavy Things: I keep 8 lb, 5 lb, and 3 lb hand weights at home. (Some of you can probably handle higher weight.) I will either do my own routine, or I will watch a five- to ten-minute YouTube exercise video that guides me through a hand-weight workout. You will be amazed at the results you can achieve after only five to ten minutes! There are so many free workout videos available online within various exercise disciplines. You don't need money and you don't need to leave the house in order to get in a great yoga, Pilates, cardio, abs, or weight-bearing session. You can also use your own body weight by doing exercises like push-ups, planks, and pull-ups.

Thoughts on Lifting Heavy Things

Building and maintaining muscle not only provides strength, but also assists with fat burning. Before digging into the details about lifting or lowering anything, it is important to address a common fear that exercising with heavy things makes women look like men. The best way to address this fear is to understand our biology. Everyone has a gene called GDF-8, and that controls a substance called myostatin, which controls the amount of muscle we have and how much muscles develop naturally. The base levels of myostatin and muscle in basically all women and most men make it impossible for them to "naturally build" bulky muscles. It does not matter how much resistance we use or what form of exercise.

Muscle size is akin to how muscle speed works. Few people are fast because few people have "fast genes." No matter how much most people run, they will never get faster than their genes will allow. However, the people who have the genetics for speed, will naturally be faster than most people (without ever training). Similarly, few people can become bulky because few people—particularly women—have "bulky genes." No matter how much most people resistance train, they will never develop more muscle than their genes allow.

You want to develop and maintain your agility, power, strength, and a great appearance? Then you want to burn fat while maintaining (or even building upon) your existing muscle. Even if you're mostly interested in burning fat, you need the muscle. Muscle is hungry. It craves protein and fat to run effectively, along with a bit of glycogen every now and then to fuel up. Next to the major organs and the brain, your muscle mass is one of the biggest consumers of energy in the body, and the more you have, the better your fat loss. It's a great cycle: the right kind of exercise spares muscle and burns fat, and more muscle with reduced body fat allows you to do the right kind of exercise.

Other Fun: I love to stand-up paddle on oceans and lakes. When I can find someone to join me, I love shooting hoops on a basketball court or engaging in a lively game of badminton or ping pong.

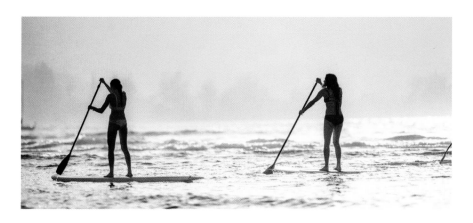

Paleo/Primal Top Misconceptions and Objections

If our ancestors' diet was so healthy, why did they all die young? I heard the average life-span for our hunter-gatherer ancestors was thirty-four years old!

This is the most common objection and misconception. First of all, let's look at the term "average." When we factor in all the deaths that occurred during childbirth, that alone significantly reduces the average life-span of our ancestors, but there are other factors involved in the average number. For example, if a hunter-gatherer man scraped his leg and it became infected, he had no chance of survival. Same goes for the hunter-gather woman attacked by a lion; there was no nearby emergency facility for that chick! The truth is, once our ancestors made it past puberty, there was a strong chance for a long life, and they lived well into their eighties and nineties.

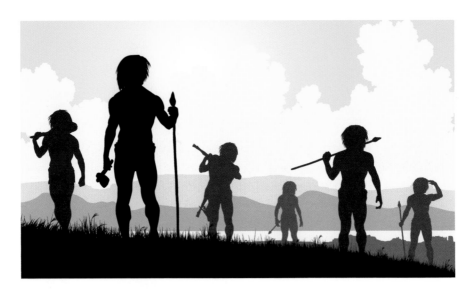

A paleo eating strategy is "high protein."

No, it is not. If we look at the overall ratio of food on any given day, paleo/primal is a high-fat, moderate-protein, and low-carbohydrate eating strategy. Overeating protein can cause gluconeogenesis, a process by which the body turns excess protein into glucose. This can be helpful if you are a hunter-gath-

erer with only animals available to consume and you need to replenish glycogen stores. It can also be helpful if you are eating very few carbohydrates and want to overindulge in protein in order for it to act as a "slow-release" glucose mechanism for you. In general though, overeating protein is a mistake many newbies make when they first adopt a paleo lifestyle. I myself was guilty of this error at first, until I made adjustments and found the proper protein threshold for me. If I decide to overeat protein (which I sometimes do), I make sure that my carbohydrate levels are even lower than normal (for me) that day.

Eating paleo/primal leads to bad cholesterol health and can cause heart disease/heart attacks.
If I had a nickel for every time I heard this! Here is my standard answer: Yes, saturated fat and fat in general can become a problem, but only if: (a) you consume it in the presence of a high-carbohydrate diet, or (b) you chronically eat way more fat than you burn. If your diet is high fat in the presence of high carbohydrates, your body will be too busy trying to deal with the excess glucose as its first line of attack; the fat will not be burned/used properly and can go elsewhere, causing problems. In fact, anyone interested in improving their cholesterol/lipid profile should absolutely adopt a paleo/primal lifestyle!

I hear from paleo devotees that they can go without food for extended periods of time when they become fat adapted. I can't do that because I have hypoglycemia, and I have to eat every couple of hours.
If you have hypoglycemia, that means you are a serious sugar-burner, and the way to manage and then ultimately get rid of hypoglycemia is to adopt a low-carbohydrate paleo/primal lifestyle. Hypoglycemia is intertwined with carbohydrate consumption, blood sugar spikes, and the adrenal glands' response to both of these by outputting cortisol. A high carbohydrate, non-paleo lifestyle is what caused you to become a sugar-burning hypoglycemic in the first place. It is reversible through lifestyle choices.

I could never quit grains because I can't go without my favorite lasagna dish (or my favorite cherry pie).
I have heard this so many times, and I find it to be such a cop-out. First of all, do you really eat that lasagna or cherry pie every day, or even every week?

*Or do you only make it a few times a year? Going paleo is not a life-sentence of **never** eating the foods you once loved. Go ahead and make your cherry pie and lasagna a few times a year and enjoy it. But stop making excuses for not going full-force into adopting a paleo lifestyle aligned with your DNA. Oftentimes, the foods that you could never imagine giving up become very unappealing after living a paleo lifestyle. Your favorite foods may change, and if they don't, go ahead and occasionally splurge on your favorite grain-based food like lasagna. That said, you should strive to eliminate those foods entirely at the onset of transitioning to a paleo lifestyle and stay the course for three to six months before deciding to indulge in something that doesn't align with our DNA map. Just know that when you do consume these foods, they should be considered fun not food. If you have Hashimoto's or any immune-based problem triggered by grains, you should consider cheating very rarely and/or switching to a paleo version of your favorite cheat meal. There are grain-free pizzas, grain-free crackers, grain-free pastas, grain-free granolas, and grain-free breads available these days, which makes it easier to stay on the paleo path.*

Whole-Life Paleo

The diet and exercise components of the Paleo Thyroid Solution will help you balance your insulin production, lose weight, and nourish your body. But if those are the only changes you make, you're going to be missing out on one of the most important pieces of the paleo puzzle— and it is especially critical to healthy thyroid function.

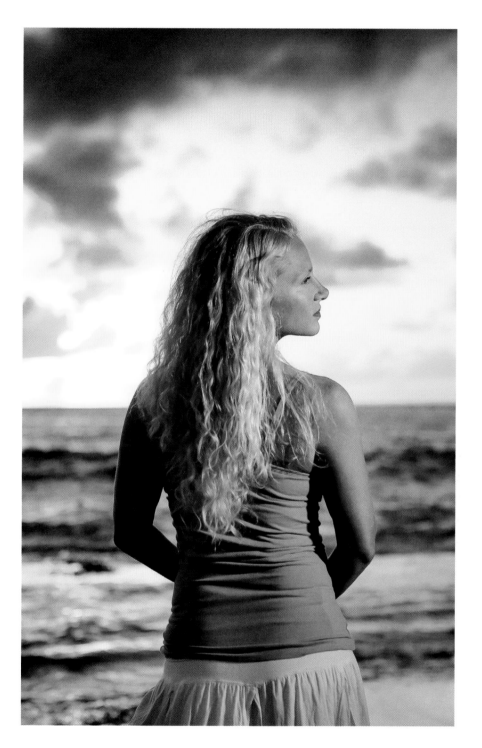

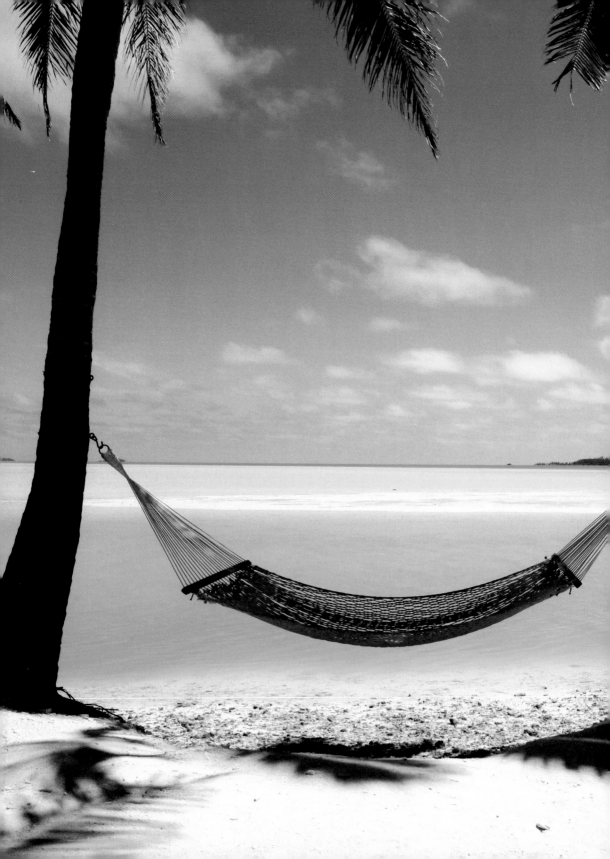

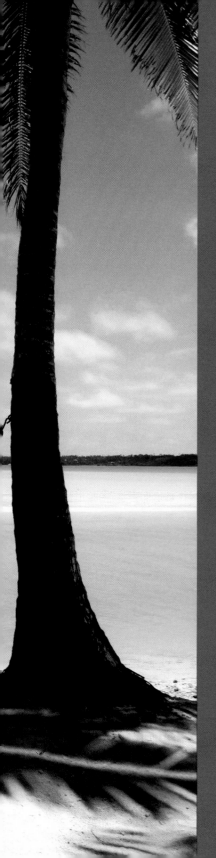

CHAPTER SIX

Paleo Lifestyle and Stress Management

Sometimes people think of stress as something negative, or they equate it with feeling overwhelmed. Not all stress manifests itself in obvious forms, and if you feel as if you don't really have any stress in your life (which is how I once regarded my life), you still might be operating under hidden stress factors and stressful activities. Stress, in all forms—obvious or otherwise—deeply affects thyroid function and overall health.

Adrenal Glands and Their Essential Bodily Functions

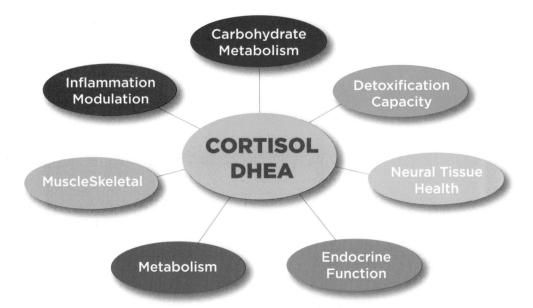

At some point in our lives, we've all been told to "just relax"; especially if you're dealing with chronic illness, you've probably heard from doctors that it's important to get enough rest. But in our insanely busy world, this can seem like condescending or impossible advice—and no one ever explains *how* you're supposed to suddenly be relaxed, or *why* it's so important. Well, the lifestyle and stress management components of the Paleo Thyroid Solution will cover the "how," and before we get to that, we need to understand *why* stress is such a big deal—not just to our mood, but to our bodies—down to a cellular level.

How Your Paleolithic Genes Deal with Stress

Faced with a stressful situation, we either get aggressive or we bolt. Our response depends upon our perception of the circumstances and our corresponding judgment of the odds of success. The fight-or-flight response is, in terms of energy preservation, tremendously efficient. And it is very effective at ensuring greater odds of survival. This makes sense to everyone on a visceral level, but let's examine the physiological mechanisms involved. The fight-or-flight response begins in the brain. Various regions operate in concert to detect, sense, decode, and respond to a stimulus. Though there are a few different pathways for a given feeling to travel (such as fear), the hypothalamus is ultimately responsible for triggering the fight-or-flight response. Once your hypothalamus goes to work, your survival systems kick into gear: the nervous system and the adrenalcortical system.

PHYSICAL SYMPTOMS OF THE STRESS RESPONSE

You are now extraordinarily alert, but only on the issue at hand—concentration and awareness of anything else fly out the window—and you may be experiencing sweating, heart palpitations, muscle tension, and/or acute hearing. The nervous system has flooded your body with adrenaline (scientists often refer to this as epinephrine) and noradrenaline (norepinephrine). Meanwhile, the adrenocortical system (which produces these hormones) becomes activated by way of the pituitary gland. The pituitary gland secretes a hormone known as ACTH, or adrenocorticotropic hormone, (say that three times fast). ACTH journeys, via the bloodstream, to your adrenal cortex, where these small organs will pump out as many as thirty different hormones to address the stressful situation at hand (the adrenals are "fed" by cholesterol). And your immune system temporarily shuts down so your body can utilize all its resources to deal with the perceived threat.

The adrenal cortex produces cortisol, DHEA, estrogen, and testosterone, among many other hormones. It's an elegant system. Unfortunately, what worked for our primal ancestors doesn't translate to working as well in our modern lives. Our modern lifestyle subjects us to a potentially enormous amount of daily stress that the body has simply not evolved to handle. Theoretically then, persistent, low-level stress, which the body unfortunately interprets as warranting a fight-or-flight response, is destructive to our health and to optimal thyroid hormone metabolism. In other words, being stuck in traffic for two hours a day, every day, is translated by your primal body as the equivalent of a serious survival threat—and the adrenals pump accordingly. Cortisol serves many important functions, including the rapid release of glycogen stores for immediate energy. But persistent cortisol release requires that other vital mechanisms effectively shut down: immunity, digestion, healthy endocrine and hormone function, and so on. The link between elevated cortisol and weight gain has already been established.

Cortisol Explained

Cortisol, a hormone belonging to the glucocorticoid family, plays a prominent role in the fight-or-flight response, as well as the functioning of nearly every organ and tissue in the body. Cortisol is produced in the pituitary gland and released by the adrenal glands in response to all stress stimulation. The fight-or-flight response can occur irrespective of whether the stimulation is negative or positive (i.e., the adrenal glands can interpret a both hectic workday and a wedding day as high-stress experiences).

Healthy levels of cortisol support the regulation of energy levels and metabolic function in the body. Cortisol is critical to the mobilization of fatty acids, glucose, and amino acids for use as energy. A crucial component of the fight-or-flight response is cortisol triggering the process of gluconeogenesis—the conversion of amino acids (either ingested or stored in lean tissue) into glucose for quick energy. In essence, cortisol is a catalyst for peak performance as it increases alertness, heart rate, blood pressure, and fuel mobilization.

Cortisol is also often discussed in the context of excess or chronic production and its destructive effects on the body. Chronically elevated cortisol from tapping into a fight-or-flight peak performance state too often, for too long, and with insufficient rest and recovery, suppresses immune function, has a catabolic effect on lean tissue, and accelerates the storage of fat, particularly in the abdomen (where cortisol receptors that promote fat storage are more concentrated). Chronically high levels of cortisol are believed to increase appetite, particularly for sugar and carbohydrates, by influencing levels of appetite hormones, such as leptin, corticotropin-releasing hormone (CRH), and neuropeptide Y (NPY). Chronically high cortisol can also result in high blood pressure and, due to sugar cravings and gluconeogenesis, a state of hyperglycemia (high blood sugar).

Cortisol levels peak in the early morning, influenced by sunlight in the human circadian rhythm, to help prepare for the stress/stimulation of the day. Cortisol levels diminish in the evening, allowing the sleep-inducing hormone melatonin to rise in the bloodstream and facilitate a smooth, relaxing transition from an alert state into a deep, restful sleep.

CORTISOL AND STRESS

Since neither burnout nor hyperarousal is desired, it's essential to understand the mechanisms of the fight-or-flight response and manage them according to genetic expectations, (i.e., to avoid chronic stressors that trigger prolonged and excessive cortisol production). Instead, life should feature occasional brief, high-intensity, intermittent stressors that serve to make us stronger and more resilient to future stress. This includes not only the obvious athletic example of conducting brief, intense workouts, but also challenging the mind with peak performance tasks (speaking in public, excelling in school or in the workplace, pursuing challenging creative hobbies such as learning a musical instrument or foreign language), and balancing all manner of stress and stimulation with sufficient rest and cognitive downtime.

Chronic Fight-or-Flight Response Drawbacks

Physical Reaction	Long-Term Impact
Blood pressure rises ⟶	Heart disease
Stress hormone rises ⟶	Anxiety, insomnia, adrenal imbalances, weight gain
Digestive system slows ⟶	Gastrointestinal problems
Growth and sex hormones fail ⟶	Accelerated aging
Immune system weakens ⟶	Infections, cancer

While it seems as though we have little or no control over our nervous system when the stress response kicks in (sure, it's hard to relax when a bear is chasing you), the truth is that we do have a certain level of control over how and when the stress response is activated during non-life-threatening circumstances. The scientific components of the stress response are three-fold. First, we have the *stimulus*, or stressor, from the environment. This could be encountering a bear in the woods, lowering into the starting blocks for a sprint race, getting into an argument with a hostile driver after a fender bender, or hearing your name called to come to the front of a packed theater for a public speaking engagement. Second, we have the individual's *perception* of the stimulus. For example, a seasoned public speaker called to deliver yet another speech will have a different perception of the event than a novice who has felt nervous and anxious about the occasion for weeks in advance. The final component is the individual's *response* to the stimulus on a biochemical level—the flood of stress hormones into the bloodstream that characterizes the fight-or-flight response.

In our example, the novice public speaker might experience a massive flood of stress hormones into the bloodstream as soon as his name is called, causing a quick spike in heart rate, blood pressure, and respiration. Meanwhile, the seasoned pro might have little or no change in biochemistry, perhaps just a slight uptick in cortisol, adrenaline, and glucose to promote optimal cognitive performance. Here, we have the exact same environmental stimulus but a different perception between individuals and a different biochemical response.

It follows that you have a choice in how you perceive stimulus, which will then directly impact your physiological response to this stress. Encountering a hostile driver can either send you into a tailspin of anger and anxiety that ruins your day for hours afterward, or it can be perceived as an opportunity to hone your skills of patience, empathetic communication, and problem-solving by remaining calm in the face of this particular environmental stimulus. When we are able to reframe our perception of an environmental stimulus, more control is gained over the involuntary chemical/hormonal elements of the stress response.

This is especially apparent when we realize that even our thoughts can serve as stressful stimuli and elicit a corresponding hormonal response. Walking alone down a perfectly benign dark alley can quickly become frightening should one's mind wander into a fearful scenario.

The health ramifications of chronic stress responses can result in adrenal fatigue, daily compromised immunity, continuous stress hormone release, feeling "on edge," exhausted sex hormones, weight gain, and compromised thyroid hormone metabolism.

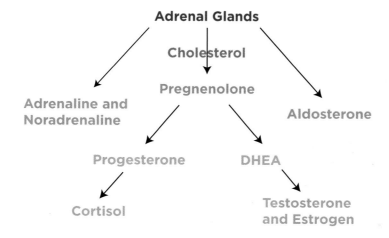

When your cortisol surges, you respond by noticing what it's paired with. It could be low blood sugar, or the scent of danger, or social isolation. Life experience builds myriad circuits that light up when your cortisol turns on. Sometimes the solution is obvious, like pulling your hand off a hot stove. But often, you're not sure what triggered the alarm. You don't know how to make it stop, yet it feels like something awful will happen if you don't "do something" immediately. For example, let's say you have a bad feeling about your boss while sitting at your desk in your office. You want to make that feeling go away because cortisol annoys you until you do something to make it stop. But you're not sure what started it or how you can relieve it. You do know, from life experience, that doughnuts make you feel good.

Doughnuts trigger happy chemicals because fat and sugar are scarce in nature. The good feeling distracts you from the bad feeling, which makes it seem like the threat is gone for the moments you are eating the doughnut. Consciously, you know the doughnut hasn't fixed your problems, but happy chemicals are molecules that pave a neural pathway. The next time you feel bad about your boss, electricity trickles to the thought of eating a doughnut. If you eat one, you build the connection. You still know the doughnut doesn't solve your problem and in fact could make it worse. But going with the flow gives you a sense of safety for that moment. When the "do something" feeling strikes, your brain builds the idea that eating a doughnut is doing something.

—Loretta Graziano Breuning,
author of *Habits of a Happy Brain*

Symptoms of Adrenal Fatigue

- Inability to handle stress
- Cravings for salty foods
- Increased energy levels in the evening (usually after 6:00 p.m.)
- Difficulty getting out of bed in the morning despite a long night's sleep
- High levels of fatigue throughout the day
- Flu-like symptoms or "I just don't feel well"
- Weakened immune system, more colds/flus and allergies worsen
- Gaining weight, especially around the waist/abdomen
- Lower sex drive
- Light-headed or dizzy when rising rapidly from a seated position or lying down
- Feelings of graying or blacking out
- Muscle weakness/soreness
- Decreased cognitive abilities
- Decreased tolerance, easily annoyed or agitated
- Increased PMS symptoms for women

- Not as productive at work or home
- Overwhelmed by small tasks
- Sensitivity to smells and sounds
- Sensitivity to light

The Importance of Sleep

Although sleep is one of the most important factors of all in managing stress and living a paleo lifestyle, this section will be relatively short. Because there's not much to say. Sleep: get a lot of it. If you're having trouble getting the requisite seven to nine hours, follow these tips for sleeping more:

- Keep your evening houselights dim and use an app like f.lux to minimize blue light on your device.
- Keep the same bedtime every night, preferably before 10:30 p.m.
- Don't engage in stressful media, conversations, or situations in the hours before you go to sleep.
- Keep your bedroom dark.

If you follow good sleep hygiene and it's still not enough, look into whether you have any nutritional deficiencies that could be interfering. Magnesium can be beneficial for sleep. If magnesium doesn't do the job, you can discuss with your doctor the use of 5-hydroxytryptophan (5-HTP). This supplement is a naturally occurring chemical in the body and is a building block to serotonin, which is a neurotransmitter that helps moderate the transmission of signals between nerve cells, and 5-HTP has been used to help raise serotonin levels in the brain. Serotonin helps regulate mood and behavior, so 5-HTP may have a positive effect on sleep, mood, anxiety, and even appetite/sugar cravings. Although 5-HTP is not found in the foods we eat and tryptophan is, eating foods with tryptophan does not increase 5-HTP levels very much.

Your entire health journey is going to be tougher and longer if you're not getting enough sleep. And sleeplessness in and of itself is a major stressor! Prioritize sleep!

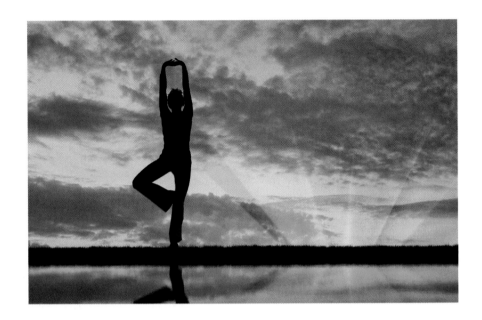

Stress: Managing Our Perceptions

It is important to realize that your body is trying to protect you at all times and save you from danger, both internally and externally. Sometimes when a person gets diagnosed with a disease or a health issue, the tendency is to see their body as an enemy. I encourage you to eliminate this perspective as you start your healing journey. Whether you just barely evaded a car accident, received a phone call with bad news, are rushing to work every morning because you're always late or you only got five hours of sleep for the past month because you've been in go-go-go mode, trying to finish your graduate school dissertation, your primal body doesn't understand the difference between a *real* threat and a *perceived* threat. Your body can react to a phone call from a negative friend griping about their day the same way it would react to you seeing a mountain lion on a hiking trail.

You might be thinking to yourself, "Elle, it's easy to suggest that I can change my reactions and perceptions of stressful events, but disappointing things happen in life: family members die, car accidents happen, money problems happen, divorce happens, etc., and you expect me to not react emotionally to these scenarios?" Not exactly. While I realize we don't always have control over our *initial* reactions and emotional responses to upsets in life, we do have control over and can prevent a spiral and continuation of the same response, by limiting how often we relive a negative experience in our minds and with our words.

For example, how many friends and family members do you call and have the same conversation about the argument you got into with your coworker last week? Do you just call one friend, vent, and move on, or do you talk about it five different times with five different people over the course of the week following the argument? Every single time you relive and retell an upsetting event or story, you are igniting those negative emotions you felt when the actual event occurred. Your body doesn't know the difference between your reaction to the *actual* event at the time it occurred and your reaction to the replaying/retelling of the event. The bottom line is your body is constantly reacting to your emotional state, which triggers hormones to become active in the body. So every time you get charged up and tell the story about that argument with your coworker, your body releases stress hormones.

In a quest for validation from others for being on the right side of the argument, or even a sense of justice or revenge you might feel by bad-mouthing that coworker to five different people, you are only hurting yourself, *physiologically*. And let's think about that for a second: you are allowing this (annoying) coworker to negatively affect your health! They are not doing it to you; you are doing it to *yourself*.

> "Low-energy words, particularly words that have a negative emotional association such as sadness or guilt, resonate at a lower frequency. They make you feel less than great by literally lowering your energy levels. In fact, 20 percent of the words you use have strong emotional undertones, which cause you to react either negatively or positively.
>
> Did you know that being happy adds nine years to your life? It has been scientifically proven that low-energy thoughts lower the immune system and make people more illness-prone."
>
> —Yvonne Oswald, PhD, author of *Every Word Has Power*

To end the spiral of focus on negative incidences and behaviors that we all come up against in life, we must dedicate ourselves to self-inquiry and self-inventory in order to gain control over of our thoughts, words, and reactions/emotions. I personally know how difficult it is to keep a positive attitude when low levels of thyroid hormones prevent your brain from functioning optimally. When I experienced my first bout of hypothyroidism and had no idea what was wrong with me, I didn't have the tools or the knowledge to even seek out books on positive thinking, the power of our words, and the power of the subconscious mind. After I recovered from the first bout of hypothyroidism, I learned about and adopted these philosophies, and my life has been amazing ever since! Those who know me well would say that I am one of the happiest, most enthusiastic people they have ever met.

After learning these tools, my life got better and better as each year went by, and I also grew happier and happier. By the time I was hit with a Reverse T3 problem, I not only had the previous success of overcoming a health challenge under my belt, but also I had the psychological and spiritual tools to help me through the depressing and physically painful process that is Reverse T3 hypothyroidism. Honestly, I still cried every day because I felt horrible in my body in every moment and my brain was not functioning properly, but spiritual audiobooks, meditation CDs on health and wellness, and podcasts were my best friends throughout my second challenge with hypothyroidism; they helped me tremendously. When things would get really bad and it seemed there was no hope on the horizon, I would say to myself, "You fixed this once already, you will find an answer, you will get to the bottom of this, and you will feel great again, it will just take some patience. But you will prevail." Contrast that with my first bout of hypothyroidism, before I knew about positive thinking and affirmation, when I would focus on negative questions and thoughts such as, "Why is this happening to me? Why am I cursed? What did I do wrong in my life to deserve this? Why won't anyone help me?" That's a dramatic difference!

Incidences of Reverse T3 and autoimmunity issues are on the rise. We must learn about and understand the nuances of adrenal health and the fight-or-flight response, because what you might *think* may not be a stressful event, your body could *perceive* as one. Adopting the paleo/primal principles on food and lifestyle is the ultimate way to adapt to the modern world by supporting the underlying causes of adrenal/stress issues. Becoming fat adapted insures that blood glucose management leads to insulin sensitivity and furthermore won't elicit responses from your adrenal glands in outputting cortisol when blood sugar drops up and down throughout the day (as it would in the instance of being a sugar-burner). When you have large fluctuations of blood glucose, your adrenal glands respond to that as a stress in the body and will rush to help you with that stress by releasing adrenal hormones.

So, if our thoughts and perceptions about our reality (e.g., reacting to a phone call from a nasty ex-husband or reacting to the loss of a job) can be misinterpreted by the body as a "stressful event"—then it follows that we should try our best to think and act in a way that continually sends the following message to our body, "You are safe." This might be easier said than done, but in our modern world of a million online resources for positive thinking, meditation, relaxation CDs, hypnosis, etc., it is absolutely achievable. When dealing with Hashimoto's-related issues and/or a Reverse T3 problem, I feel it's important to *thank your body for trying to protect you* and to view your body as an ally versus an enemy on your path to wellness. Connecting your mind and body in this way can make a world of difference in your healing journey.

On a psychological and spiritual note, a common theme among patients with thyroid issues is the inability to speak up (or not having a voice in a situation), including the inability to express oneself creatively. For my entire life, I've rarely had issues speaking up about anything; everyone who knows me would laugh at the thought of me not speaking my mind. My mother raised me to speak my mind and to not let anyone patronize me. I generally have very high self-esteem and self-worth.

Although I never had issues with speaking up in other areas of my life, I had issues speaking up in romantic relationships—until hypothyroidism showed up in my life. Before then, I often found myself in relationships where I didn't feel I had a voice, and I would get that choked-up feeling in my throat. After discovering and tuning into this personal nuance, if I felt choked up, I took serious inventory of the relationship and looked at what I may or may not be expressing. Thankfully, through a lot of audiobooks, life coaching, self-inquiry, and self-inventory, I ended the pattern of attracting relationships where I put myself in a position of not having a voice.

Everyone reading this book has likely experienced a fight-or-flight adrenal response. Whether you were watching an intense thriller film where a bad guy popped out of nowhere with a knife or you spotted a mountain lion on your hiking trail, we can all relate to the shaky/alert feeling running through our veins that is sparked by our adrenal glands when we visually, or mentally, perceive a threat.

How you perceive events in life will dictate your adrenal responses. It's important to know your thoughts get translated into emotions, and those combined can spark hormonal responses in your body. When those hormonal responses are chronically negative, they contribute to the overload and subsequent exhaustion of your adrenal glands.

Self-Inquiry, Visualization, and Coaching

I became aware of the power of positive thinking after solving my first bout of hypothyroidism. So when a Reverse T3 problem showed up, I actively filled my life with audiobooks, podcast interviews, and films related to spiritual healing, the power of positive thinking, and the power of the subconscious mind. While I am a fan of many authors who write on these subjects, there is one resource that comes to mind as a must-see for anyone struggling with a health issue. The movie *You Can Heal Your Life,* based on Louise Hay's book, was released right at the time I was hit with a Reverse T3 problem. It was a game-changer for me and instilled in me hope and practical ideas about how to look at my health issue and life in general. If you are experiencing hypothyroid symptoms currently, then you may know how hard it is to read, focus, and comprehend words on a page. I found that listening to audiobooks or watching films and interviews was the only way I could receive and retain information at the time.

I think it is essential to avoid watching dramatic, depressive, and/or negative TV shows and films while you are trying to heal a health issue. I found it helpful and uplifting to watch and listen to comedy and positive stories about people's health transformations. Look, there are plenty of people who have it worse than you do now and they were able to solve their health crisis; listening to success stories of healing can ignite the hope and desire necessary to get through a health crisis.

Make a vision board to hang in your house, or make a smaller version that you can keep private if you don't want others in the household to see it. Devote the entire vision board to health and healing; it can be a continual source of inspiration and hope while also imprinting your subconscious mind with positive health affirmations every time you see it. I always have a few vision boards in my house. I also have an artist's sketchbook that I fill with magazine clippings of things I want to have or achieve in life; sketchbooks are great because they are easy to take in a backpack or stow away when company comes over. You can paste old photos of yourself when you used to be fit and in shape on the vision board or paste photos from fitness magazines of bodies that you find attractive—inspirational reminders of what is possible. Below is an example of a healing vision board.

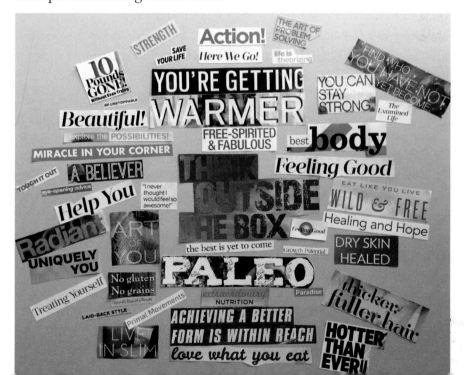

I am a devoted fan of HayHouse.com and its associated free online radio station, Hay House Radio (also a free smartphone app). At all hours of the day on Hay House Radio, there are shows hosted by authors, healers, and life coaches spanning all subjects related to mental, physical, and spiritual health. Gaia.com is also a favorite. They offer online monthly paid subscriptions with access to hundreds of spiritual and scientific videos, movies, lectures, interviews, and many exercise/yoga videos.

Another invaluable resource is life coaching; it helped me immensely. Most life coaches offer a free twenty- to thirty-minute consultation over the phone. And even though I am a paleo/thyroid coach and life coach, sometimes coaches need coaching! But many years before I became a coach myself, I searched for a life coach online. I had free phone consultations with three different life coaches; two women and one man. Honestly, from the start I assumed I would likely go with one of the women coaches, but I did not resonate with either of them. In contrast, I was blown away by the consultation I had with the male life coach and chose him.

These days, I coach myself the majority of the time, but occasionally a coach needs another coach to help them gain perspective on something they might be blind to. Jeffrey Brownstein (Shine@LifePurposeU.com) has been my life coach since 2007 and has been an amazing addition to my life. On average, I speak with Jeff about twice a year now, whereas when I first started coaching with him, I spoke with him once a month and sometimes more. (The wonderful thing about life coaching is that it can be accomplished over the phone.) It's important to find the right coach for *you* and hire someone *you* resonate with. I continually strive to be the best coach I can be for my clients, but my personality and coaching style may not click with everyone. And this holds true for any coach.

From my experience in dealing with two separate bouts of hypothyroidism, I can say that what saved my sanity the second time around was the fact that I had been sick once before and overcame it. Previous experience told me my symptoms were temporary and fixable. It is really difficult when you are experiencing hypothyroidism for the first time to imagine a day when you will feel totally normal, happy, vibrantly healthy, and excited about your future. At first, it feels as if it's never going to get better. But just like with relationships, once you have healed from the heartache of a romantic breakup, the next time around may be a little easier, because previous experience assures you that a breakup is not the end of the world; you will carry on.

If you are experiencing hypothyroidism for the first time, just know that it is *fixable*. Once people start on the correct thyroid hormone replacement and get all of the other components in order, they start to feel better four to six weeks after starting thyroid hormones, and it can take six months to a year for all the hypothyroid symptoms to disappear—not that long in the grand scheme of a long life. You have the highest chance of success if you dedicate yourself to learning all that you can about hypothyroidism while adopting a paleo/primal eating and lifestyle strategy to support your goals.

Relationships and Career

Hypothyroidism can negatively affect relationships of all kinds: Work relationships, romantic relationships, family relationships, and friendships. One of the toughest things about hypothyroidism, is that people can't see a lot of the symptoms versus seeing someone in an arm-cast or a wheelchair, so it's hard for them to comprehend and relate. People seem to be more sympathetic to ailments they can visually identify.

Some hypothyroid patients get fired from their jobs, experience divorce or separation, and even lose friends and family members over the condition. I had several problems with family members and friends when I was very sick with undiagnosed hypothyroidism—I didn't know what was happening to me. A year after I started NDT and was feeling great, my best friend called, choked up with tears, to apologize. He admitted that he thought I was just being lazy and a spoil-sport during the time I was hypothyroid. He said he had felt annoyed and resentful of my lack of interest in participating in fun things and being social. After he saw me go through my thyroid journey and understood the situation, he felt terrible, because he realized my behavior wasn't really "me." It wasn't my choice to be exhausted and unsocial.

Family members, friends, coworkers, employers, and significant others need to understand the perils of hypothyroidism. Most people with hypothyroidism are physically and mentally exhausted. They need help at home cooking, cleaning, and running errands; even the slightest chore can be overwhelming and stressful for someone with hypothyroidism and adrenal issues. And once you know that you have hypothyroidism, it's important to share your diagnosis and the symptoms with loved ones, and in some cases, your boss. Hypothyroid patients often become less productive at work and are unable to complete tasks and solve problems in the same efficient manner they once used to.

People in your life need to know that hypothyroidism is fixable, and that it might take six months to a year, which requires patience from everyone. And ask for *help*! Six months to a year is not a long time in the grand scheme of life to rely on others for assistance with things you temporarily cannot do.

A MESSAGE TO THOSE DEALING WITH A HYPOTHYROID PATIENT

If someone in your life has just been diagnosed with hypothyroidism, you have to understand that any questionable behavior on their behalf is not who they truly are nor how they are choosing to be. If you read this book, you will realize why this is the case on a physiological level. But even if you're reading only this section because a loved one handed you this book, you need to know it is imperative that the person in your life suffering with thyroid issues gets ample rest and, as much as humanly possible, is not confronted with stressful situations.

If you live with someone suffering from hypothyroidism, this is the time to step up and help out around the house why they heal themselves, which can take six months to a year. It's important to understand that any depression experienced by the hypothyroid patient, combined with any erratic or annoying behavior, is somewhat uncontrollable on a biological level; personality issues can go hand in hand with hypothyroidism because of how the brain is affected. While I am not excusing or condoning bad behavior, you need to know that hypothyroidism (or hyperthyroidism) can bring out the worst in people's personalities. Most of all, it is important to know that this will not always be the case! Since many patients are undiagnosed for long periods of time, it may be tough to believe that your loved one will have a 180° transformation, but they truly can. When your loved one fixes the problem naturally or gets optimized on thyroid hormone replacement, their behavior and overall disposition will change for the better in every way. In the meantime, however, they need your patience, your help, and your support.

If you employ someone suffering from hypothyroidism, it's important to be patient and understand that your employee will step back up to the same level of productivity they displayed before hypothyroidism. Because cognitive function and energy levels are negatively affected by low levels of thyroid hormones, your employee might have an impaired mental ability to process certain tasks at the same speed, and it might take them longer to complete a task. If your business allows, it would be extremely helpful to your employee to temporarily reduce their workload, and if possible, reduce the amount of time they spend at the office, perhaps even allowing them to work from home a few days a week or take a paid sabbatical.

It's hard not to resent or be angry with someone who snaps at you, is unable to comprehend you, forgets things, is easily agitated, stressed out, and offended, and is generally no fun to hang out with. Hypothyroid patients can also become extremely sensitive to noises, sounds, and smells. It's essential that you understand these types of behaviors and sensitive reactions are very common among the millions of people suffering from hypothyroidism.

Remember, people are usually not themselves while suffering from hypothyroidism. Your hypothyroid loved one, friend, or employee needs your *help*, not your *judgment*. They will change for the better as their thyroid condition gets resolved. Support them in getting there!

A MESSAGE TO HYPOTHYROID PATIENTS

Of course, it's not your fault that you have hypothyroidism or that hypothyroidism altered your brain and body chemistry in such a way that your personality changed and you started treating others poorly. However, I think it's wise to apologize for your behavior and to explain to others what is happening. If you have lost or become alienated from friends or family members (or are fearful of losing your job) you have to understand everyone else's position: they are probably unaware of what is happening in your body, so they may assume your personality issues are who you have become. You should have compassion for them, just as they should have compassion for you.

If you want to repair a relationship that fell to the wayside or was negatively affected by your hypothyroid state, then take responsibility for the situation by acknowledging your behavior and thoroughly explaining the changes taking place in you. Share excerpts from books and online resources that explain how low levels of thyroid hormones and adrenal issues affect the brain, cause depression, and can turn a person anxious, easily agitated, impatient, and intolerant. Apologize and assure the people around you it won't be long before you are back to normal. And let them know that, until then, you need their support and understanding.

Stressful Solutions

I just spent a whole chapter telling you to find ways to decrease the stress in your life. But maybe tackling thyroid disease feels too stressful in and of itself (which it can be, and I have been there!). That's why, in the next chapter, I lay out in step-by-step detail how to implement the Paleo Thyroid Solution to help you avoid feeling overwhelmed and stay on track.

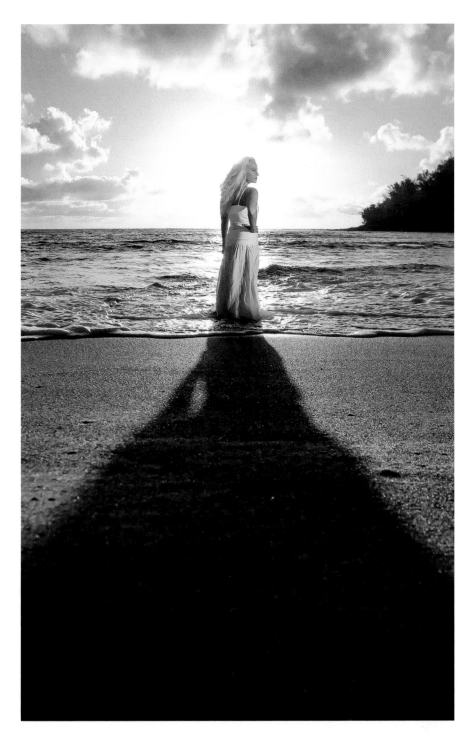

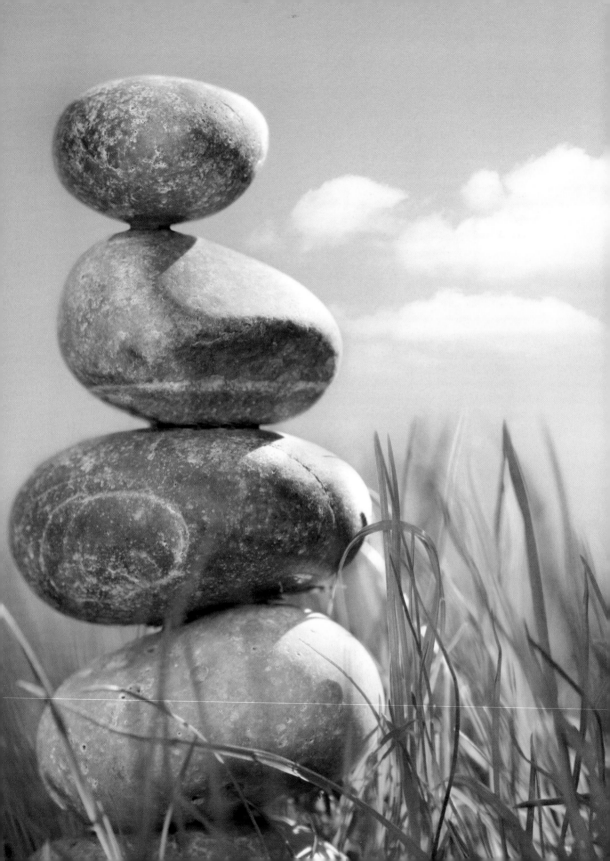

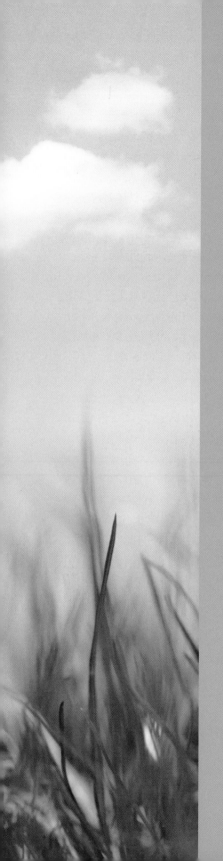

CHAPTER SEVEN

Implementing the Paleo Thyroid Solution

The minute you stop improving yourself is the minute your life becomes stale. Never stop challenging yourself to become the best you can be.

—Mo Seetubtim,
*founder of The Happiness Planner
and BrandMentalist*

Now that you are armed with information to start your journey, can you really dive into all of this at once? The answer is, probably not! I've laid out some phases for you to implement the Paleo Thyroid Solution while optimizing your health and respecting your body's delicate hormone balance.

Phase 1

If you are currently hypothyroid and have not yet fixed the problem naturally, or if you have not yet reached thyroid hormone replacement optimization, then your body is not functioning at an optimal level necessary to adopt *all* the principles involved with paleo/primal living (like intermittent fasting, sprinting, and more intense strength training). However, you can start by adopting the basics to begin detoxifying your body, assisting in recovering adrenal function, and balancing your blood sugar levels (all of which contribute to thyroid hormone metabolism). While you might not lose a significant amount of weight during Phase 1 due to lingering thyroid and adrenal issues, you can start the process of healing the underlying culprits of thyroid dysfunction while also training your body to become fat adapted.

You can stay in this phase for as long as it takes to get optimized on thyroid hormone replacement and/or resolve nutrient issues. If you are attempting to resolve thyroid issues naturally (without thyroid hormones) using the Paleo Thyroid Solution, give yourself twelve to sixteen weeks, minimum, of *strict* adherence to Phase 1 before retesting thyroid and nutrient levels.

In Phase 1, focus on these strategies:
- Work on optimizing your hormone replacement dosage.
- Eat paleo foods.
- Stay under 150 total grams of carbohydrates per day
- *No* exercise or *extremely light* exercise (i.e., relaxed, short walks or very simple, easy yoga).
- Start applicable supplements.
- Sleep and nap as needed.
- Manage stress.

Phase 2

If you have been in Phase 1 for a while and have noticed dramatic improvements in your energy, overall health, and/or improved lab results, you are ready for Phase 2. Whether you are reversing a thyroid issue naturally (or have started thyroid hormone replacement and are close to being optimized), you can start to adopt more paleo strategies as your energy increases and symptoms disappear.

In Phase 2, focus on these strategies:

- Stay under 150 total grams of carbohydrates per day.
- Primary exercise, namely walking.
- Lift heavy things once a week.
- Try fasting once a week.
- Keep up with supplements.
- Sleep and nap when needed.
- Manage stress.

Phase 3

If you have finally resolved your thyroid issues by following Phases 1 and 2, or if you are optimized on thyroid hormone replacement with the elimination of most or all of your symptoms, you are ready to adopt all the paleo lifestyle principles.

In Phase 3, focus on these strategies:

- Stay under 150 grams of carbohydrates per day but experiment to find your personal carbohydrate tolerance level. If you are insulin resistant or have not achieved significant weight loss, start with dropping down to 80 grams of carbohydrates per day and adjust up or down from there. On a personal note, I don't feel good when I eat more than 70 grams of carbohydrates per day. I feel even better when I am below 50 grams per day and in ketosis (more on that in Phase 4).
- Weekly sprinting session or other high-intensity exercise once a week (i.e., tennis, advanced yoga, aerobics, crossfit, etc.).
- Lift heavy things two to three times a week.

- Fast one or more times per week.
- Keep up with supplements.
- Manage stress.
- Once you have reached this phase, you probably won't find daily naps necessary, but take a nap anytime it's needed, and make sure you're still prioritizing your nighttime sleep.

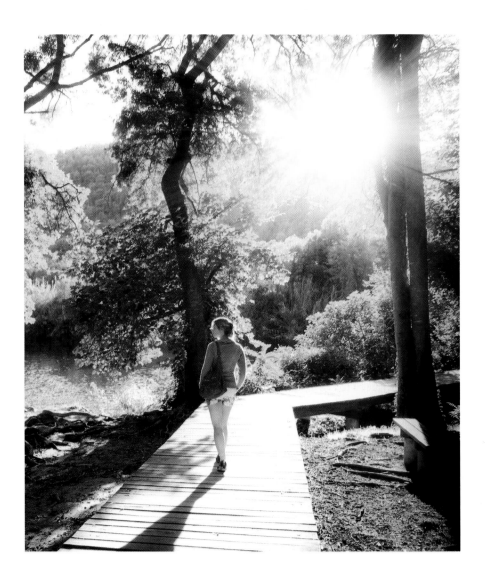

Phase 4

Burn lingering, excess body fat with nutritional ketosis! Once your thyroid health is in order and you've been fat adapted for a while and feeling good, ketosis can be attempted if you feel that you are still not burning fat efficiently. Sometimes hypothyroidism leads to a state of insulin resistance or even type 2 diabetes (happened to me), but both are completely reversible through carbohydrate management. In my case, I had to go extremely low carbohydrate in order to zap excess stubborn fat on my body that I had gained during my two bouts of hypothyroidism, and it took me awhile to reach that conclusion. I realized that I had become very carbohydrate-intolerant and so I experimented with going lower and lower with carbohydrate consumption; I not only started to burn fat, I felt mentally and physically better all-around.

What is *ketosis*? Ketones are compounds created by the body when it burns fat stores for energy. When you consume a diet very low in carbohydrates, the body responds to the significantly lowered levels of blood sugar by flipping the switch to another power source. The body converts fatty acids in the liver to ketones. For many people, this switch can be flipped when adhering to 50 grams of carbohydrates per day, but for some people, going down to between 20 and 25 grams of carbohydrates per day (or still lower for some people) is necessary in order to ignite the fat-burning metabolic machinery.

Ketones, then, become the main energy source as long as blood sugar levels remain low. *Ketosis was crucial to our evolution.* Given the relatively minor role of carbohydrates (even the consumption of many tubers is thought to have come later, with the advent of cooking practices), our ancestors' bodies were frequently operating under ketosis. Considering the fasts and famines of primal living, it is clear that ketones served as an essential energy source.

For anyone attempting to drop below 50 grams of carbohydrates per day, it's important that you fully research and study the nuances necessary to successfully achieve and stay in ketosis. For example, more salt intake is needed in the diet when one is in ketosis, consuming more fat is essential, and sometimes lowering protein intake is key. For anyone interested in learning all about the nuances involved in nutritional ketosis, I recommend the following resources, all of which were essential in my journey.

- *The Art and Science of Low Carbohydrate Living* by Jeff S. Volek, PhD, RD & Stephen D. Phinney, MD, PhD
- *Keto Clarity* by Jimmy Moore with Eric C. Westman, MD
- *The Livin' La Vida Low-Carb Show* with Jimmy Moore (free podcast)
- *Low-Carb Conversations* with Jimmy Moore, Jenna the Paleo PA & Friends (free podcast)

I've Tried Everything but I'm still Having Issues!

If you have adopted all of the tools available in this book, and you still feel as though something is "off," whether it is not being able to lose weight or you are experiencing any other lingering symptoms, below is a detailed list of things to investigate further. You can also try these avenues while you follow the protocols in this book for a very comprehensive approach.

FOOD SENSITIVITIES AND FOOD ALLERGIES

Sometimes it's obvious when a food affects you negatively because you feel it. However, sometimes certain foods can cause inflammation or other problems systemically without manifesting through obvious symptoms. Taking a food sensitivity test (like ALCAT) can reveal these hidden factors. When I had lingering weight-loss issues and inflammation (revealed through blood work), I took a food sensitivity test and discovered that I had a severe intolerance to cocoa. I had been eating dark chocolate and cocoa powder, sometimes daily, until taking that test! These tests reveal sensitivities ranging from foods/herbs to chemicals and preservatives and could help you resolve lingering symptoms and issues.

HBA1C TEST

In chapter 3 I mentioned this insulin sensitivity/diabetes screening blood test. If after adhering to a strict paleo regimen for a while you don't see the weight-loss results you want, insulin resistance or type 2 diabetes could be the culprit, and both are reversible through a very low-carb eating strategy. For people without diabetes, the normal range for the HbA1c test is between 4% and 5.6%. Hemoglobin A1c levels between 5.7% and 6.4% indicate insulin resistance (or just too much carb consumption) and an increased risk of type 2 diabetes, and levels of 6.5% or higher indicates diabetes. While mainstream medicine might suggest that a result of 5.7% is considered normal, Dr. Foresman suggests that an HbA1c result over 5.2% is a major red flag and anyone with a result over 5.2% should take a serious look at their carbohydrate/sugar consumption.

CANDIDA

Candida is a fungus, which is a form of yeast, and a very small amount of it lives in your mouth and intestines. The healthy bacteria in your gut typically keep your candida levels in check, but sometimes it takes more than just strict adherence to a paleo lifestyle to get rid of it. Candida assists with nutrient absorption and digestion, when present in normal levels. When it overproduces, if left unchecked, it breaks down the walls of the intestinal lining and penetrates the bloodstream. This releases toxins from your system, causing leaky gut syndrome. Symptoms can include brain fog, trouble with weight loss, hormone imbalance, loss of sex drive, chronic sinus issues, bad breath, gas and bloating, and more.

Changing up your probiotics every month along with the conservative use of oregano oil can assist with clearing up candida issues. I myself had candida issues without knowing; it was revealed only after getting tested by Dr. Foresman. I suspect it was left over from my former sugar/grain addiction days combined with my two bouts of hypothyroidism. Because some of the candida symptoms are similar to hypothyroid and low iron symptoms, I think candida is important to get assessed and under control as soon as possible, so you can correctly gauge what is truly causing symptoms that mimic hypothyroidism. Candida, like all fungal issues, is encouraged and "fed" by sugar in all forms.

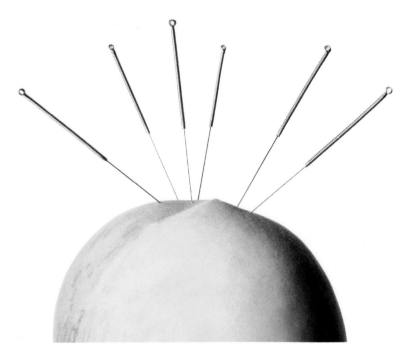

CHIROPRACTORS/ACUPUNCTURISTS

I have seen situations where people's thyroid issues were completely *revealed and fixed* through chiropractic visits and/or acupuncture visits. If you wish to try to resolve thyroid issues naturally first, before going on thyroid hormones, then living a strict paleo/primal lifestyle along with trying alternative therapies can attack the problem on a variety of natural levels and might offer the best chance of success at resolving hypothyroidism in a natural way.

Other Avenues

- Explore systemic enzymes (not *digestive* enzymes) for inflammation, estrogen dominance, fibrocystic breasts, fibroids, scar tissue, and high levels of fibrinogen in the blood. (The use of systemic enzymes alleviated hidden inflammation for me and completely resolved my painful, fibrocystic breasts and brought my fibrinogen levels back to normal).
- Consider high-dose vitamin C for inflammation.

- Investigate alpha-lipoic acid (ALA) supplement for blood sugar issues/insulin resistance.
- Consider an organic acids urine test that looks at biomarkers from various metabolic pathways. These biomarkers give an overview of several major systems in the body and an analysis of nutritional deficiencies in the body. (My candida issues, for instance, were partially revealed through this test, along with low levels of serotonin and vitamin C.)

Changing Unhealthy Patterns

"When you are not taking actions that you feel you need to be taking, or when you are taking actions that are in conflict with your values, there is often a tremendous drain on your sense of wholeness and well-being. Smoking is a good example of this for many people. Even though they may not even have said that they were going to quit, usually people are at odds with themselves for continuing to engage in an addiction that they know is doing them harm. There is an inconsistency in the self and therefore, one is in a weakened state."

—Katherine Woodward Thomas, author of
Calling in "The One": 7 Weeks to Attract the Love of Your Life

For many years I was a cigarette smoker and a sugar/food addict. I overcame both addictions through willpower and a paleo lifestyle, but not without substantial planning ahead for the transition. Giving up an addiction is like giving up an important part of who you are and how you think. No one can convince you that you are out of sync with your personal goals—only you can. I probably would have continued to smoke if, deep down, I hadn't felt bad about myself every time I lit up a cigarette. I knew I was essentially contributing to an early death every time I smoked, and that created a lot of inner turmoil. On the one hand, I was making green smoothies, taking supplements, and working out to *improve* my health, while on the other hand, I was canceling out those efforts every time I smoked a cigarette. I was a walking contradiction: I would finish a two-hour hike and immediately light up a cigarette afterwards. For some people, quitting grains, dairy, or sugar is like quitting smoking—they cannot imagine life without it. There was a time I could not imagine life without cigarettes or grains, but my cravings for them are gone, and I see them both for what they truly are: poison for humans.

When you are full-force in the midst of an addiction of any kind that addiction becomes your best friend, your crutch, and your comfort. If you are currently addicted to food, or think about food a lot, it's very hard to hear people in the paleo/primal communities talk about how little food they get away with eating, because to a food addict, eating *less* food sounds horrible! The thought arises, "But I don't *want* to eat less food. I *like* eating a lot of food. I wish I could eat *more* food!" I truly, wholeheartedly understand this conundrum, and I am here to tell you that once you get over the hump of being a sugar-burner and transition into being a fat-burning warrior, you will look back and feel so sad for your former, addicted self. You will shake your head, laugh to yourself, and think, "Wow, I can't believe what a slave I was to food and how obsessed I used to be. I wish I knew about paleo/primal living years ago."

In all sincerity, it only takes four to six weeks of strictly adhering to a paleo/primal lifestyle to reverse a lifetime of food obsessions and addictions (assuming underlying factors such as thyroid hormone levels and nutrient levels are optimized). What is six weeks in the grand scheme of a long life? Planning ahead is important. If you love grains, then perhaps a cold turkey strategy won't work well for you. Go ahead, enjoy all the grains you want, while planning ahead and choosing a date when you will start your primal journey and get rid of the grains in your life once and for all. After four to six weeks of strictly adhering to a primal lifestyle (and doing it correctly), you won't look at grains the same way again. The positive changes in how you feel and look will dictate your disdain for the tasteless, gooey, glucose-filled, antinutrient poison that is grains.

SAY NO TO SCALES

I avoid scales at all costs when focusing on fat/weight loss. Let's be honest with ourselves, we know how we feel and look in our own bodies, and we do not need a scale to tell us whether or not we are on track; all we need is a mirror and clothes. Often, weighing yourself or even looking into a full-length mirror (especially when you are not happy with your body) can be a major downer, because it can act as a negative reminder of not achieving your goal yet.

Do yourself a favor by focusing on living a paleo lifestyle and becoming an expert at intuitively figuring out what your own body's nutritional needs are. You will *see* and *feel* the results. When I was miserably hypothyroid and living in a bloated, fat body, one doctor weighed me at 155 lbs (I am 5'2"). I cried for days after that appointment, I had never been that heavy in my entire life. I was mortified. I already knew that I was overweight, but seeing the number made it even worse!

After that experience, I never weighed myself, and at future doctor's appointments I would instruct the nurse to not tell me my weight result. I would stand on the scale backwards while the nurse weighed me, and I would ask them to put the scale back down to zero after we were done, so that I wouldn't accidentally catch a glimpse of my weight. If you are insistent on weighing yourself, do so after you have already felt significant changes in your body and after you have noticed that your clothes are getting looser. After that benchmark, you could weigh yourself again, after you've noticed further changes, and so on. When you finally feel *awesome* in your own body, weigh yourself a final time to get a baseline snapshot of what your weight is when you feel your best. Or don't weight yourself ever again—your choice!

SAY YES TO CLOTHES

You will feel the inspiration and success of adopting a paleo lifestyle when your clothes start fitting you differently, or not fitting at all because they are too big! When I was at my heaviest, I could not pull my size 26 jeans up past my calf muscles! It was a horribly depressing moment to say the least—I felt like an adult trying to fit into children's jeans—and I was mortified. I kept those jeans around for years because I knew that someday I would be able to get back into them, and I wanted to experience that. I cried tears of joy on the day I finally felt ready to try on those jeans again, and they slipped right up my body with ease. In fact, they were loose and I needed to drop down to a size 25 jeans (hurray!).

Did I need a scale to gauge my success? Not at all. Use your clothes as success indicators and stay away from the scales until you feel amazing in your own body. When you feel and look great in your body, it won't matter what the scale says. And at that point, weighing yourself can be fun and educational, to see what your body fat percentage is along with your weight to determine a baseline for when you feel and look your best.

You Can Do This!

With every step you take on the Paleo Thyroid Solution path, you will be healing your body and coming closer to optimum health. My coaching clients have been where you might be right now: sick, tired, overweight, stressed, lonely, and dealing with doctors who just don't understand. By following the phases laid out in this chapter, they have achieved remarkable improvements in their health—read about some of them in the next chapter. I know you can achieve the same success!

CHAPTER EIGHT

Thyroid Success Stories

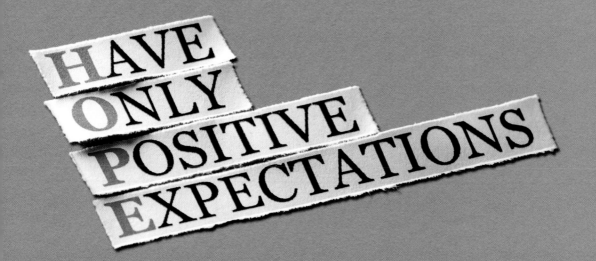

When I was at my worst, I often despaired of ever feeling better. I had no idea whether I would be able to resolve my health issues, and I knew very few people who had successfully navigated the difficult terrain of trying to get good, knowledgeable thyroid treatment. So for you, the reader, who may be in the same frightening, ill place I once was—someone who doesn't really know if she'll ever feel like herself again and who cannot find a doctor to trust—I've included this chapter. These stories are to give you hope, to inspire you to keep searching for answers, to know that others have walked this difficult path and emerged into a life of health, vitality, and happiness. Read them as many times as necessary to help you along the way.

My Story

The first indication that something was wrong with me was in 2003, at the age of thirty, when I started my period two weeks early. Since I had experienced normal gynecological health all my life until this point, I didn't consider it alarming, and I figured it was a fluke. I finally went to the doctor when I started bleeding again just two weeks later, and I was having worse than usual menstrual cramps. I went to my doctor and his immediate response to my symptoms was to put me on the birth control pill in order to control the bleeding (which is a classic solution, in my experience, from uninformed doctors).

My entire journey of suffering from hypothyroidism could have been avoided at this point, had my doctor asked the question, "What is causing this healthy, fit thirty-year-old with perfect gynecological history to start bleeding abnormally?" Unfortunately, my doctor did not ask this question (and neither did I). Instead, he continued to prescribe a variety of birth control pills, each one stronger than the last, because they all kept failing to control the abnormal, excessive bleeding. But I trusted my doctor's advice—a mistake. Throughout the many months I tried the various birth control pills he prescribed, I rapidly gained weight and constantly felt as though I was in a bloated, menstrual state. This made no sense because I exercised regularly, and I had what most people would consider a fit physique. I am 5'2", I was 110–115 lbs, 16% to 17% body fat, and before hypothyroidism hit me, I exemplified the image of health and fitness.

Someone suggested to me that I might have a thyroid problem, so I went back to my doctor to have him test my thyroid–another big mistake. Here was a doctor who didn't even think to inquire about the root cause of my bleeding, and here I was trusting him to take appropriate blood tests. Yikes! In retrospect, that should have been a major red flag. My doctor tested my thyroid incorrectly by only testing my TSH. He said the TSH was within range, I did not have a thyroid problem, and I just needed to exercise more and eat less, which I thought was impossible because I had been working out two hours a day and eating 1,200 calories or less; yet, I was continuing to gain weight.. He looked me in the eye and told me, "Well, it's *not* your thyroid." Had this doctor been knowledgeable enough to test my Free T3 and Free T4 levels at the time, he would have concluded that it was in fact my thyroid—I was seriously hypothyroid—and I might have been spared the horrendous experience of full-blown hypothyroidism. It took me two years from this point to get diagnosed properly.

My symptoms progressively worsened. I was freezing all the time, even in hot weather; my temperature was 96°F versus the normal 98.6°F. I was exhausted and very depressed. I started to get acne, even though I had flawless skin my entire life. I was unknowingly very anemic with restless legs; I was bloated, heavy, and miserable in every way with constant menstrual bleeding and cramping. Life was horrific, and I barely left my apartment. I cried multiple times a day; I could hardly stand being in my own skin. I had zero control over my body and symptoms. I kept going to doctors who continued to tell me that there was nothing wrong with my thyroid.

One of the worst moments during this time was on a hike with a friend, I started to experience such severe abdominal cramps that I thought I had to take an emergency bowel movement. I walked into the woods, took down my pants, assumed the squat position, and huge blood clots fell out of my vagina onto the ground. I write this with tears in my eyes, recalling how frightened and horrified I was about my future. It was one of the scariest days of my life.

After the incident, I saw a gynecologist who misdiagnosed me with PCOS. Did I have PCOS? *No and sort of.* My state of hypothyroidism threw off all of my sex hormones so drastically that my pelvic ultrasound looked like the classic profile of someone with PCOS (there were sixteen or so cysts in a ring around one of my ovaries). This scenario is a perfect example of why anybody with a gynecological problem or low levels of sex hormones needs to get their thyroid tested accurately. Because the thyroid is the master gland affecting every system in our body, including our hormone levels, a state of hypothyroidism can lead to something else that will become a disease the person *wouldn't have gotten otherwise.* My hypothyroid state eventually led to the formation of a polyp on the lining of my uterus and also a uterine fibroid. Because the polyp was on the lining of my uterus, it kept poking the lining and making it impossible to stay intact, which caused more bleeding and constant vaginal leakage (not cool!)—ultimately leading to severe anemia. And my depression only got worse.

I went to so many doctors and spent thousands of dollars on specialized MDs who didn't take insurance—some were famous authors and hormone doctors to Hollywood celebrities. At some point along the way, you would think a doctor would have questioned my iron levels based on the amount of bleeding I was experiencing from my gynecological issues, but no one did. Finally, there was one doctor who tested my Free T3 and Free T4. It cost me $600 for that office visit (not including labs) to have a doctor finally test my thyroid *correctly.* I was relieved to know, at last, that a thyroid problem was causing all of my health and weight issues.

Below are the thyroid labs that took me *two years*, thousands of dollars, and an insane number of doctor's visits to have a physician finally declare, "You are very hypothyroid."

ELLE—NOVEMBER 2005 *(Hypothyroid Diagnosis)*

TEST	RESULT	RANGE	NOTES
Free T3	1.52	(1.80–4.20)	*below* the range
Free T4	1.28	(.80–1.90)	
TSH	1.08	(.40–4.00)	

As the above values show, if an endocrinologist had tested just my Free T4 and TSH (which many endocrinologists do), they might have concluded, "Your thyroid looks fine." These labs show how critical Free T3 testing is. This horrifically low level of Free T3 directly corresponded with every symptom I was suffering from. I retested six weeks later, to see if things were still the same, before starting thyroid hormone replacement.

ELLE—JANUARY 2006

TEST	RESULT	RANGE	NOTES
Free T3	2.86	(2.30–4.20)	not below the range, but low
Free T4	.075	(.80–2.30)	below the range
TSH	1.56	(.50–5.50)	

After this two-year journey, I was not only broke but also disheartened by so many doctors *hurting*, not helping me. So I began to search the internet 24/7 to find answers. Life had ground to a halt, and my days were filled with physical misery, existing in a state of disease that I could not control. The only advantage I had in my quest was that I worked from home and was able to rest when I needed to. I had gained more than 40 lbs, and that was with exercising daily. (In retrospect, exercise was something I should not have been doing.) Thankfully, my internet searching led me to learn about ferritin and how essential it is. I got tested and my ferritin was 10 in a range of 10–150, which meant I was severely anemic and had restless legs. I learned that if I didn't improve my iron levels, no amount of NDT was going to help me, and I would face difficulties raising my NDT dosages, which would halt my progress.

At this point in my journey, I could not afford any more doctor's visits, but based on my experience with doctors leading me in the wrong direction, testing me incorrectly, and misdiagnosing me, I also did not trust them to solve my hypothyroidism. So, I took my health into my own hands and started down the path of treating my own hypothyroidism with NDT—without the help or the assistance of doctors. I relied solely upon my own research and intuition, combined with the advice and wisdom of fellow patients from patient-to-patient online chat groups.

In January 2006, just six weeks after seeing my low levels of T3 and ferritin, I started taking iron. I simultaneously started taking NDT. I started to feel improvements a couple of weeks later: my restless legs started to subside, my heart palpitations began to dissipate, I had more energy, and my brain function started to kick back in. After a couple of months on NDT and iron, I was feeling better and better as every day passed. After a full year on NDT, my hypothyroid symptoms vanished and life returned to normal. I also had surgery to remove the polyp from my uterus lining, and soon after the surgery all of my gynecological issues were completely resolved. I was feeling normal again! I spent the next six to seven years on NDT feeling wonderful (although I still felt obsessed with food and found it a struggle to maintain my weight loss, because I had not yet discovered paleo/primal living). During those years on NDT, whenever I cried, it was out of gratitude for finally feeling like a normal human being again! *Yeah for NDT!*

UNTIL 2011

In 2011 I began to feel the onset of hypothyroid symptoms: Inability to keep off weight, rapidly gaining fat around my stomach area and waist, dry cracked skin, inability to focus, brain fog, and depression. You might assume that because I previously experienced the perils of hypothyroidism that I would recognize hypothyroid symptoms right away, but I didn't even consider it. I had been living well on NDT for many years until this point, so it seemed impossible that my symptoms could be related to thyroid.

My symptoms got worse, really fast. My hair was falling out and felt rubbery to the touch. I started to get very constipated and bloated. I was exhausted no matter what I did or how much I slept. I was overwhelmed by small tasks, and became extremely sensitive to light, sound, and smells. My face was puffy every morning. My legs were heavy and bloated. I can't even recall how many times I sobbed in the shower; I was washing a bloated, fat body that was foreign to me. I would even cry on the toilet…I had gained so much weight that I struggled to reach back to wipe myself (a horrible experience to say the least). The weight gain and bloat seemed even *worse* than the first bout of hypothyroidism. Depression came back with a vengeance.

I went to a doctor, who I had found after getting myself optimized on NDT. Even though I had successfully treated myself for years without the aid of doctors, during my six to seven years on NDT, I kept searching for a doctor to *legitimize* what I had been doing without one. About three years in to taking NDT, I found what I was looking for. Not only was this doctor impressed with my story of self-treatment, but also I was able to educate her about the importance of ferritin (which she was unaware of), and she began implementing ferritin tests with her other thyroid patients. I thought I had scored the coolest doctor on planet Earth! A doctor who listened, wanted to help me, wanted to learn, and was confirming my own strategies? Jackpot! I finally felt "legit" about my thyroid treatment and health. As you might imagine, I referred a lot of people to this doctor. I trusted her, because when I first met her, she was open and willing to admit that she didn't know everything about thyroid health. She also seemed to understand NDT dosing and was not worried about my suppressed TSH.

Well, after experiencing the second onslaught of severe hypothyroid symptoms, I went to see that doctor. I was a bloated, fat mess sitting across from her as she scanned her clipboard, "Your blood tests, your thyroid tests . . . they all look great. I don't know what to tell you about the weight gain and brain fog." And then she proceeded to give me exercise and nutritional advice that fell on deaf ears (I was already exercising and restricting calories). I evaluated my blood results too. From what I could see, my labs looked normal, but I noticed that the T4 was higher than usual. At the time, I didn't know this was a red flag. I left her office confused about what was causing my symptoms. A myriad of hypothyroid symptoms came crashing down on me after that; it was so severe that I didn't feel as if I was on thyroid hormones at all! I felt just as terrible as I did before I was diagnosed many years prior. Except this time, I experienced no abnormal menstrual bleeding. Like my doctor, I too eliminated the possibility of my symptoms being related to thyroid, but I was determined to find out what was wrong with me. The fear of possibly getting another gynecological problem drove me to research my situation 24/7 again, and I eventually suspected that I might have a Reverse T3 problem.

I went back to my doctor and asked her to test Reverse T3 along with Free T3, TSH, and Free T4. She didn't understand Reverse T3 but she ordered the tests for me anyway. The blood results proved my suspicion, I was experiencing a major Reverse T3 problem. I went back to see my doctor with a folder packed with research on the subject and plans for how to fix it. I explained to her how I had reached the diagnosis and told her that I wanted to take T3-only to fix my Reverse T3 problem. She looked at me, very annoyed, shook her head and said, "Oh Elle, this is just too complicated."

I felt so betrayed and angry in that moment. I started sobbing. I stood up and said, "Let me show you something." I stripped down to my underwear and stood in front of her. I had gained so much weight that my bra barely covered my nipples—it resembled a very skimpy bikini top that a Playboy bunny would wear to a pool party.

"Look at me. I'm *huge*! I keep gaining weight, I can't think, I'm depressed, I'm exhausted, and I have all the other classic signs of hypothyroidism, dry cracked skin, skin thickening. I am seriously hypo-thyroid right now! This is *too complicated*? But medical school wasn't *complicated*? Organic chemistry problems on the MCAT were not *too complicated*, but *this* is too *complicated*!? Please help me! I need help!"

She looked at me as if I were crazy. "I'm sorry I can't help you with this, but I will try to find someone who can, and I'll have my office call you with a referral." (I never got a referral even after calling the office three more times.)

Below is my blood work from when I was on NDT but had developed an RT3 problem and had become severely hypothyroid a second time, because the T4 in my NDT was being converted into the biologically inactive Reverse T3. As you can see, my Free T3 is high and could poten-tially look normal for someone on NDT (except that I had hypothyroid symptoms). My high Free T4 was a red-flag indicator that I might be experiencing a major Reverse T3 problem. The ratio between my Free T3 and Reverse T3 confirmed that I did indeed have an RT3 problem.

ELLE—JULY 2011 *(Reverse T3)*

TEST	RESULT	RANGE	NOTES
Free T3	4.2	(2.3–4.2)	
Free T4	1.7	(0.8–1.8)	
TSH	1.56	0.01	"suppressed"
RT3	33	(11–32)	
RT3 Ratio: 12.7			

Free T3/Reverse T3 Ratio: 20 or higher is considered healthy.

I walked out of the doctor's office and sat in my car, sobbing. Here I was again, in the same position as I had been seven years prior, when no one in the medical community would help me. I felt so alone in that moment, because I had a gut feeling that I was going to be on my own again for the second time with hypothyroidism. My gut feeling was confirmed when, after *pleading* with thyroid specialists and doctors in Los Angeles to help me, not one of them would. The vast majority of the medical community was, and still is, clueless about diagnosing and treating Reverse T3, especially with T3-only.

The doctors I spoke with were very afraid of T3 for no apparent valid reasons. Not one MD I spoke with prescribed T3 without T4 to their patients, and most of them warned me that T3 was very dangerous and that I could give myself a heart attack. I didn't believe them. I started doing a ton of research on T3 and Reverse T3 and discovered an online group dedicated to the subject, which I joined. I received amazing emotional support and invaluable advice. After learning about the myths surrounding fears that doctors have of using T3-only, I became confident that T3 was not going to kill me. In fact, I became quite confident that T3 would accomplish the opposite—T3 would *save* my life. It did. And it still does.

Because I had the luxury of working from home, I was able to closely monitor my blood pressure, pulse, temperatures, and symptoms without worrying about onlookers. I took detailed notes on everything I did and everything I felt. It took about ten weeks to start feeling normal again, but I still struggled to lose the excess weight I had gained.

After sixteen months on T3-only, I finally adopted a paleo/primal lifestyle. I knew I had discovered something unique when not only the weight started falling off me, but I was able to reduce my T3 dose significantly. Most importantly, food addictions, food obsessions, and unhealthy cravings disappeared! I couldn't believe that. From teenage years on, I always felt a struggle with food and diet. Even though I had once achieved a body I was thrilled with before hypothyroidism entered my life, I achieved it through conventional low-fat "eat three to five meals a day" diet wisdom, and I always felt as though I had to sacrifice, suffer. And frankly, I thought it was the only way to achieve ideal body composition because every diet book I read said the same thing. When I had been on NDT, I had managed to lose most of the hypothyroid weight, but it always felt like a struggle to keep it off. I was always thinking about what I was going to have for my next meal, I was hungry every two to four hours, and I always felt I had to use extreme willpower with portion control and everything else regarding eating. I honestly felt as if I was cursed because I saw other friends and how they ate; it didn't seem as though they had the same issues with feeling obsessed with food. I could not understand why I did.

After going paleo and getting fat adapted, my former food addictions and obsessions all made perfect sense, and most importantly, they disappeared! When I strictly adhere to a paleo lifestyle, I have zero issues with food obsessions and sugar cravings. Although if I veer off course, they come back. In fact, I rarely think about food until I am hungry, whereas I used to think about food all the time! It was a relief to know that there wasn't something inherently wrong with me after all those years of struggle. I was simply eating against my genetic programming, against my DNA map. The evidence is overwhelming in favor of a paleo/primal lifestyle for keeping adrenal glands in check, managing blood glucose, and eradicating food addictions/obsessions.

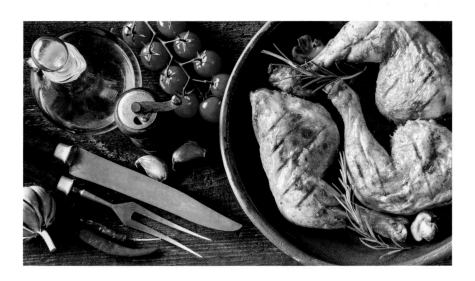

MY JOURNEY IN PICTURES

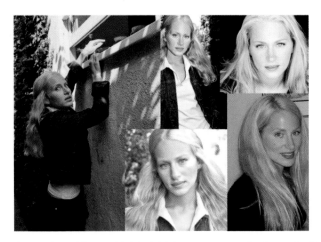

Before I got hypothyroidism (2000–2003) I was very fit, lean, feeling great in my body and averaging between 110 and 115 lbs. I was a size 2–4.

The onset of hypothyroid symptoms began in the fall of 2003. The symptomatic weight gain is especially apparent in my face in these photos from a wedding I attended in the fall of 2004. I was miserable behind that smile. I had gained more than 40 lbs, even though I was exercising one to two hours a day.

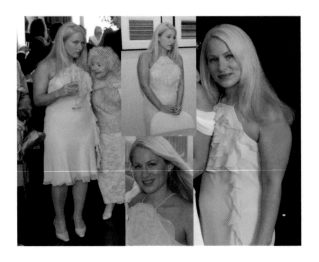

In January 2006, I started NDT, and it took about a year for me to feel good in my body again and simultaneously correct low iron and adrenal fatigue. These photos were taken between 2007 and 2010, when I was on 3–3.5 grains of NDT, which I multi-dosed twice a day. I was convinced that I had solved my hypothyroidism forever.

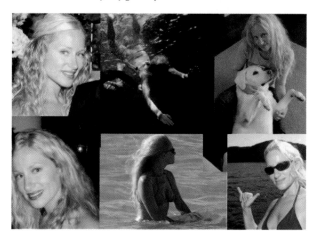

I didn't know my body was brewing an RT3 problem at the time, but this was two months before the onset of full-blown Reverse T3 hypothyroidism. I was starting to get bigger and more bloated and was having trouble keeping weight off.

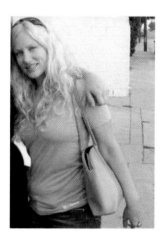

However, the photo on the right, taken July 26, 2012, is after four months on T3-only. It took me three of those four months to fix my Reverse T3 problem and feel better. In this photo, although I felt considerably better in every way, my weight had still not budged much (only 10 lbs down). I was doing hot yoga classes five to six days a week (which I later realized was chronic cardio and part of the problem).

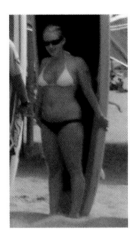

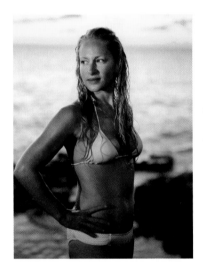

The picture to the left (taken in June 2015), is after three years on T3-only and one and a half years after going paleo.

Although I wish I hadn't gone through any of this, I am glad I did. I not only have a profound appreciation for feeling normal, but it is my hope that all of my mistakes and misdiagnoses along the way, will help other people who are worried they might never be well again.

Classic Uninformed Doctor Experience

Doctors who are uninformed about the use of T3-only are very confused when they see lab results from people on T3-only. I was visiting Kauai, in Hawaii, and as an experiment I decided to see a doctor who was considered one of the best on the island. I brought along my blood work, drawn one week prior to my arrival, to show him. First, I gave him an in-depth explanation about what happened to me over the years and why I ended up on T3-only. I also explained that I was writing a book on this subject and that I had fixed hypothyroidism on my own twice in ten years. My experiment was intended to see whether he would prescribe T3-only, so I told him that I was running out of my T3 pills and I needed four weeks' worth, to last until I flew back to the mainland. (This wasn't actually true, but I wanted to create an emergency-like situation.)

After my explanation, he said, "I wonder what the active thyroid hormone is?"

I immediately responded, "I can tell you right now it's T3. T4 is just a pro-hormone and the only biologically active thyroid hormone is T3." He wasn't going to take my word for it; he consulted his smartphone, and I reiterated, "I will bet my life that the answer is T3." His Google results ended up confirming what I had just said.

Confused, the doctor used his pen to write "TSH" on the examining table paper protector and said, "But if your TSH is zero, there is no way to tell whether or not you are on the right amount of medication."

"The TSH is an outdated test and should not be used as a measure to dose patients," I said.

"Well, that's what we do, we use the TSH to dose patients," he said.

I took his pen and began writing diagrams and making all the connections between TSH, T4, T3, and Reverse T3 to explain in detail why my TSH was suppressed and why it wasn't a problem.

He kept repeating, "But we dose based on the TSH." I told him he could look up the entire subject online and that there was plenty of evidence suggesting otherwise. I reiterated that this method of treating patients is outdated, even harmful. He didn't get it; he didn't even try to understand it.

This is a doctor regularly treating thyroid patients with thyroid hormones (T4-only and NDT), yet he has no idea what the active thyroid hormone is. Wow! Since he mentioned that he actually prescribes T3 for depression to some of his patients, I thought there might be hope that he would understand T3 and write me a prescription.

Even though the lab results I brought in were merely one week old, he insisted on testing my thyroid levels again. I assured him my labs would not change. "I am happy to get blood work done again, but I do not want to waste my time or money, because my blood work will come back looking exactly the same as you see it now. So, I need to know beforehand, will you prescribe me T3 based on these exact results? If not, then I don't want to bother taking labs."

"I have no problem prescribing you T3, but I need to redo your labs," he said.

You can probably guess how this story is going to end. I got my lab work done and the results were exactly the same as the previous week's results.

When I followed up with his nurse a few days after the results, the message I received was, "The doctor doesn't feel that you need T3."

"You are kidding me right? I am currently on T3. I live off T3, and I cannot live without T3, so I would love to know why the doctor reached this conclusion? Furthermore, I told the doctor not to waste my time and money by getting blood work done if he already knew this would be his conclusion… Instead, he wasted my time and money. To boot, I waited forty-five minutes to be seen by him."

"I think you should file a complaint," the nurse said.

After I hung up the phone I just started bawling, not because I needed the T3 prescription (I didn't), but because here was just another example of the doctors who keep patients hypothyroid due to lack of knowledge and lack of interest in learning about thyroid health; this one was still relying on the TSH test and was clueless as to what the biologically active thyroid hormone was.

The encounter only refueled my desire to get the word out about this all too common experience with doctors. Doctors routinely dismiss evidence or research that patients bring them and underestimate patients' intelligence. Doctors like these are unwilling to look further into a problem beyond their training, and they won't even entertain the notion that a patient might have something valid to contribute. In my opinion, this behavior borderlines on malpractice.

———

Hawaii is a perfect example of what happens when we divert from the genetic DNA blueprint our bodies were programmed to follow. Primitive Hawaiians did not consume grains, nor did they have an obesity epidemic as they do now. Hawaiians once lived a primal existence, consuming mainly coconut, fish, pigs, fruit, and taro. Taro, a potato-like root vegetable, can be made into taro chips or consumed in the form of poi, a mashed-up, cooked-down version that develops into a thick paste. Although taro is very starchy, Hawaiians got plenty of sunlight and exercise, along with rest and play, and any excess carbohydrates present in the taro were not enough to send them into a high-carbohydrate, sugar-burning lifestyle.

When Hawaiians lived off the land and sea, and they were fit and fierce. Until sugar cane production came to Hawaii. Later on, rice showed up and then fast-food chains. In present-day Hawaii, unfortunately, obesity and type 2 diabetes are prevalent.

My forty-five-minute wait in the doctor's examining room in Kauai afforded me plenty of time to peruse the various informational posters hanging on the walls. After my disappointing discussion about thyroid health with the doctor, I pointed out the same posters, illustrated below.

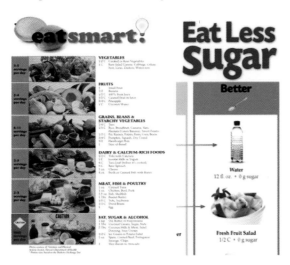

I said to the doctor, "This 'eat smart' poster is telling people to eat six to eleven servings of grains a day on top of two to four servings of fruit, which constitutes a diet high in carbohydrates and which we know promotes type 2 diabetes. Yet, this information is coming directly from the government food pyramid. So, do you as a doctor believe the government is right?"

He smirked and shook his head no.

"Well then, I have some questions. First of all, why do you have this poster hanging on your wall? This information is misleading patients and hurting their health by promoting a high-carbohydrate, pro-inflammatory, and pro-type 2 diabetes diet. Secondly, if the government is saying that six to eleven servings of grains per day is considered 'healthy and smart,' but you and I both believe the government is wrong, wouldn't you be willing to accept that perhaps some of what you learned in medical school twenty to thirty years ago regarding thyroid health might also be outdated and wrong?"

He was silent.

I pointed to the second poster. "This says a bottle of water has 0 g of sugar, which is true, but then right underneath the bottle of water it states that a half cup of fresh fruit also has 0 g of sugar. This is factually incorrect. You and I both know that a half cup of fruit equals a minimum of 5 g of sugar, and anyone with an internet connection can reach the same conclusion. By displaying these on your walls, you are dispensing misinformation that contributes to the promotion of type 2 diabetes, even though the whole point of these posters is to prevent diabetes. If you know that a high-carbohydrate lifestyle like the one these posters suggest contributes to insulin resistance and type 2 diabetes, why on Earth would you be encouraging such a diet?"

The doctor just held his hands up in the air as if to say, "Oh well, that's how it goes."

I really wanted to rip those posters off of the walls and put up a warning sign: Don't see this doctor for your thyroid health! The hypocrisy, the depth of ego, and the unwillingness to learn about new developments in thyroid health and nutrition/type 2 diabetes were astounding. How many more doctors are displaying this kind of misinformation?

If the Pacific Diabetes Education Program wants to educate people about type 2 diabetes, they are doing a terrible job based on the flawed government *food pyramid, the SAD. For an in-depth look at the history and politics surrounding the current government food pyramid, check out Denise Minger's book Death by Food Pyramid: How Shoddy Science, Sketchy Politics and Shady Special Interests Have Ruined Our Health.*

Sher's Story

I developed an eating disorder when I was twelve. Fifteen years later, the anorexic, bulimic, binging behaviors had taken a serious toll on my body and my health. I gained and lost hundreds of pounds during this time and my yo-yo dieting, rapid weight gains and losses, and horribly misguided nutrition left me feeling like, well…absolute shit.

I started a stressful corporate job after college and things went downhill from there. Late nights, tons of caffeine, and chronic cardio (in an effort to "finally get my butt in gear") only did further damage to my body. For the hundredth time, I tried eating less and exercising more in an effort to lose weight. For the hundredth time, it did not work. I could not sustain the calorie restriction and exercise it took to lose and keep off weight. I would burn out, and as soon as I went back to normal calorie consumption the weight would pile back on. The more I repeated this cycle, the less it worked. Losing weight was an epic battle, and it would come back on seemingly overnight.

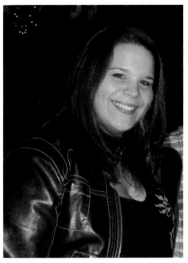

When my boyfriend (now fiancé!) introduced me to the ancestral health field (hat tips to Mark Sisson, Robb Wolf, and Angelo Coppola), the approach to nutrition seemed crazy enough to actually work, so I gave it all a try. I changed the way I thought about, bought, prepared, and ate food.

My all-time heaviest in 2011 at 220 lbs.

Food quality increased, I cut out gluten and processed foods, and I cut back on alcohol and sugar. I eliminated all but high-quality, high-fat dairy. With these changes alone, I dropped about 15 lbs.

Aside from the weight loss, which plateaued, everything else kept going downhill. As part of my corporate job, I took international assignments in both Montreal and Costa Rica. Living abroad added more stress to my life, and my inability to handle the anxiety and depression I felt meant I was overwhelmed *all* of the time. I had no energy. Sleeping ten or more hours a night left me feeling exhausted and drained. I had to set multiple alarms just to get myself up in the morning, and my caffeine intake gradually increased to boost my alertness. Getting through the week became harder and harder as my energy levels went lower and lower. My hair was so dry and brittle that it would break off in my hand when I ran my fingers through it, and it had all but stopped growing. My fingernails were thin and flimsy and ripped constantly, and my skin would be cold to the touch, even under layers of clothing.

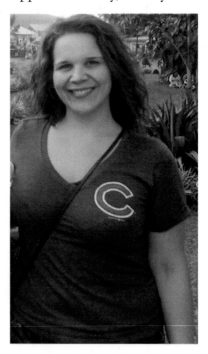

I had absolutely no endurance. Intense exercise left me with numb lips and heavy legs, and I couldn't explain why. I would drudge up the energy for a workout, but after about thirty seconds of high intensity I would have to stop. I tried to push myself through this point several times, but it resulted in seeing stars and getting dizzy. It was as if someone had completely drained my energy tank. I was thirsty all the time. My pee was clear, but drinking water didn't make me feel hydrated. Digestively, things weren't going so well either. I pooped once a week, maybe. At the age of twenty-five, I had hemorrhoids that showed up pretty

In 2012 my hair was breaking off daily and was the texture of straw.

regularly due to constipation (but this was normal for me, and at the time I didn't even recognize this as an issue).

The most acute and worrying symptoms for me were mental and cognitive. Mentally, my memory was so poor that if I didn't write down a phone number, appointment time, name, or task *immediately*, I would forget it. I asked myself daily, "What is wrong with me? Am I stupid?" My job consisted of numbers and spreadsheets, but I couldn't read them in the right order and constantly mixed up digits. Emotionally, I was anxious and depressed. I felt overwhelmed by the simplest things, and my heart rate would skyrocket with stress. It took less and less to get me worked up, and I often ended up in tears. I started getting hives as a result of the anxiety.

I went to my doctor, looking for answers, and he ran a few tests. He concluded that all was well and left me with a quick message: "You're fine. You just need to eat less and exercise more to lose the weight. Try a low-fat diet...and work on managing your stress. If you want, we can try antidepressants." It was a message I had heard before, but it didn't feel like the right answer to me anymore. I was armed with enough ancestral health knowledge at this point to know that something wasn't right.

I found a naturopathic doctor who was willing to work with me. After hearing my symptoms he said it was most likely that I was hypothyroid. We did a comprehensive blood work panel and an adrenal salivary test.

Below are the first results of my thyroid test.

SHER—APRIL 2014 *(Before starting NDT)*

TEST	RESULT	RANGE
TSH	2.77	(0.450–4.500)
Free T4	1.19	(0.82–1.77)
Free T3	2.6	(2.0–4.4)

My adrenal panel came back with pretty advanced adrenal fatigue, and a picture started to come together. After reviewing everything, the "official" diagnosis was adrenal fatigue and malnutrition from a lifelong eating disorder. What about a thyroid issue?

"No," he said, "your thyroid tests do indicate suboptimal thyroid status in my opinion, but nothing that I would deem to be abnormal." (Direct quote from an email exchange we shared.) We started a supplement regimen, and I saw some improvement to my energy levels as my adrenal glands received back-up from the adaptogens, adrenal complex, vitamins C and B12, magnesium, multivitamin, and Celtic sea salt I was taking. I quit caffeine, and things improved a bit more. My weight stayed put, and this doctor also told me that my issue was willpower related, that I should focus on eating less and exercising more (though to his credit, he did not recommend chronic cardio). I was getting pretty sick of that being the only answer, and I constantly questioned why I struggled so much against my body.

In September 2014, I met Elle at Mark Sisson's PrimalCon event, and my life was forever changed.

I overheard Elle talking to someone about her own thyroid story, and my interest was piqued. I had heard of hypothyroidism and had started doing some research about it after my own thyroid was tested, but I knew almost nothing. I approached her and explained where I was and how I felt. We spent the next couple of hours talking about thyroid and adrenal health, and why the conventional medical system so often fails hypothyroid patients. Elle told me exactly what blood tests to get, and she helped me find an NDT-friendly doctor in Chicago. We also talked about things I could do in the meantime to start supporting my adrenals and body. She truly empathized with me, and she was adamant that my situation was not hopeless and that she would help in whatever way she could to get healthy again. She was so encouraging and positive about my future, even when I could not see the silver lining.

I left California with hope, for the first time in a long time, that I could feel better.

Back in Chicago, I saw an NDT-friendly doctor and he retested everything. I took a twenty-four-hour cortisol test, and it was clear I had major cortisol/adrenal issues. The doctor wanted to treat my adrenals first to see if my thyroid function would resolve. Five months after starting adrenal supplementation, my thyroid picture didn't change much.

SHER—NOVEMBER 2014 *(Before starting NDT)*

TEST	RESULT	RANGE
TSH	3.5	(0.450–4.500)
Free T4	1.2	(0.82–1.77)
Free T3	2.4	(2.0–4.4)

My doctor agreed to start me on NDT to see how raising my levels would improve my symptoms and adrenal function. We started with 1/2 grain of NDT in November, and I gradually raised my dosage over the next several months. By May I was on 3 grains, and I was starting to see and feel massive changes in my body and my mind.

My hair started growing, and it became shiny and strong again. My nails stopped cracking. I started pooping every day (and man, that makes such a difference, especially without hemorrhoids). My memory improved. My ability to problem-solve came back. My family and friends noticed an improvement in my mood and behavior. I felt as if I could handle being social without feeling so overwhelmed (something I had attributed to becoming increasingly shy with age). I felt witty again. I started sleeping soundly for eight hours and bouncing out of bed in the morning. I started seeing an improvement in things I didn't even realize were issues. My eyelids weren't puffy in the morning anymore. My thirst level went down. My sex drive increased! And my PMS symptoms (cramping, bloating, flow, mood swings) and anxiety all decreased. While I still occasionally get hives, it is a rare occurrence these days. Weight-wise, I've lost about 10 additional pounds since May 2016. The weight has come off very gradually (and all from around my midsection), and I have changed nothing about my diet, which is a whole foods–based, gluten-free, lowish carbohydrate diet. Now that my energy is up and my endurance is back, I am able to be back in the gym, lifting weights and sprinting.

In addition to all the work that I've done to get myself physically back to health, I've also done a tremendous amount of inner work to heal the emotional eating and emotional attachment behaviors I had related to food. I even became certified as an Eating Psychology Coach to lead myself through the waters of emotional eating, and now I coach others through these waters as well. In the last two years, I have changed jobs and careers, moved, and let go of people or things in my life that caused more stress than they were worth. I decided to place my health as the first priority in my life. Now, for the first time ever, I feel like all the pieces of my health are moving in the right direction together. Progress has been slow, and I've also had to exercise patience throughout, but I am determined to keep moving forward. Elle was the missing piece for me in my confusing puzzle of mental, emotional, and physical health.

SHER—AUGUST 2015 *(Ten Months After Starting NDT)*

TEST	RESULT	RANGE
TSH	0.01	(0.450–4.500)
Free T4	1.1	(0.82–1.77)
Free T3	3.5	(2.0–4.4)

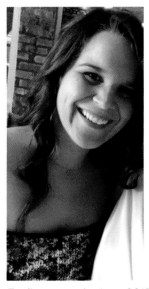

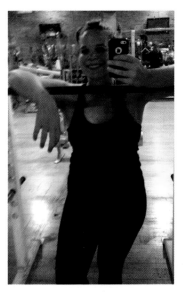

Feeling great in June 2015.

Enjoying my workouts again in September 2015.

I feel like a new person! Elle helped me understand certain tweaks in dosing and offered ideas about how and when to take my NDT to further optimize my situation. Elle has been an amazing resource along the way, supporting me on this path to better health. Without Elle believing in my story when my doctors would not, my life would be much different than it is today. I am now pregnant with my first child, weeks away from delivery, and I have gained only 17 lbs—everyone is amazed at how good I

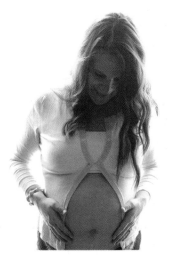

look and feel. I have lots of energy, minimal hormonal or mood swings, and stable weight. I am still exercising every day and even heavy lifting! My current NDT dose is 4 grains (2 grains in the morning and 2 grains in the afternoon), which is up from 3 grains since the start of my pregnancy. I am so happy that I feel this great! Thank you Elle!

Morgan's Story

The winter of 2012, when I was twenty-eight, I started to notice changes in my digestion: feeling super bloated every night and just generally sick after I ate. I was going to the bathroom less and less. And the constipation…ugh! Awful. I was freezing all the time, cold hands and feet. I'd lay in bed, and my butt would literally be cold to the touch. It was bizarre! I was working from home at the time, and I remember not wanting to get out of bed, I was that cold. I'd work from my bed until eleven, which was ridiculous because I live in Los Angeles and grew up in Chicago; 60°F should have seemed warm to me! I was napping every afternoon. I'm not a sleepy or lazy person: I work out every day, eat very clean, and surf three to four times a week. But during this point in my life, I was really exhausted all the time, especially at 3:00 p.m.

A few things happened right around the same time these symptoms started showing up. I gave myself a Christmas gift of an appointment with a naturopathic doctor in San Diego and had complete panels done on everything you can imagine: stool test for parasites, blood work for micronutrients, DNA analysis, etc. I took a quiz on thyroid from a book on different health conditions one may have, and concluded, I'm definitely hypothyroid.

I got my blood drawn in February, read the book in March and self-diagnosed hypothyroidism, waited a few months to get my blood work taken, do the stool test, get my blood work results back, and schedule a follow-up appointment with my ND. She confirmed my suspicion.

MORGAN—JULY 2014 *(Before Going on NDT)*

TEST	RESULT	RANGE
TSH	0.94	(1.80–3.00)
T4	4.10	(6.00–12.00)
T3	75.00	(85.00–205.00)

The values for T4 and T3 above are not "free" results because I didn't know at the time what the better tests were. You can still see that all of the results are below the range.

During this three- to four-month period, I was super stressed out, commuting three hours a day (ninety minutes each way), I gained 8 lbs in three months (which is about 8% of my body weight because I'm only 5'0"), and was getting depressed. I was eating super clean, low-carbohydrate, and so forth, but the weight would not budge. A group of my high school friends came into town for a mutual friend's bachelorette party when I was at my lowest: I didn't want to be social (which is not like me at all; I am very outgoing), and I fell asleep during their visit and woke up four hours later. Something was wrong; I am the most social person I know.

I started on 1 grain of Nature-Throid in June. By July, I quit my job. About five weeks after starting Nature-Throid and one week after quitting my job, I lost 5 pounds in one week without trying. Over the course of the next month or so, I got back to my natural maintenance weight of 99–113 lbs and I remained there effortlessly for three months. I started having bowel movements, anxiety went away, and I didn't feel stressed. I started looking good and feeling good about life.

MORGAN—SEPTEMBER 2014 *(On NDT)*

TEST	RESULT	RANGE
TSH	0.029	(0.350–5.500)
Free T4	0.96	(0.89–1.76)
Free T3	2.8	(2.3–4.2)

These results only after two months on 1 grain of NDT—I got the "frees" tested at this point, you can see the TSH getting suppressed and the Free T3 and Free T4 are moving up. I am starting to feel better at this point.

In the early months of 2015, I got lazy again. I was unsure my Nature-Throid was doing anything for me, and I stopped taking it to embark on a personal experiment to see if my own thyroid would kick back in and do its job. Really, I just didn't want to schedule an appointment and pay for more labs. And I'd switched doctors and had a bad experience with insurance. So I procrastinated over dealing with it. Simultaneously, in an attempt to get "really fit" and sculpt my arms, I started following the advice of bodybuilder trainer. I started eating carbohydrates. Well, it took all of three months and 10 lbs for me to throw my hands up in the air, text Elle, and get myself back on track. I hadn't been this heavy since my beer-guzzling, gluten-eating college days. I was distraught and my body wouldn't budge. I was constipated again, and when I did manage to go, my stool was like rock-hard pellets. Elle guided me through my options and advised me on which panels she thought I should test; lo and behold, my thyroid hormone levels were at the bottom of their ranges. So in June 2015, I went back on Nature-Throid, but this time I started with ½ grain and then increased to 1 grain in six weeks.

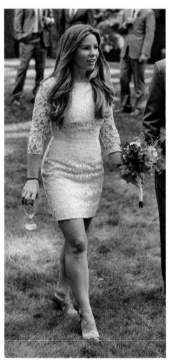

Honestly, I don't think any doctor ever had my thyroid optimized. I learned a lot in my "experiment," comparing how I feel when I'm not on Nature-Throid to how I feel when I'm on thyroid hormone replacement. There are considerable changes in almost every aspect of my life.

When I'm on Nature-Throid, my weight is naturally stable and in my maintenance range. Before going back on meds in June, my weight was going up and up and up with no end in sight, no matter how much I surfed, how cleanly I ate, or how many strength-training sessions I did during the week. As soon as I started treating my hypothyroidism, the upward spiral turned around and my weight started to come back down again. I feel more like myself. I'm a light-hearted, free-spirited goofball

Morgan feeling and looking incredible in October 2014.

again. Four weeks after I started on Nature-Throid again, I was think-ing, "This is the regular Morgan!" So much lighter and more fun! I'm sure less anxiety and depression have something to do with it. My sex drive was virtually non-existent when I was off thyroid hormones, but it came back—thank God! And I no longer nap. I have energy all day.

My diet hasn't changed, my workout routine hasn't changed, my boy-friend hasn't changed. I have a lot more energy to last the entire day than I ever did pre-diagnosis; I'm getting older, yet my energy level is increasing. I have experimented with different dosages, with my doctor, and as of right now, my current NDT dose is .75 grains, which I take first thing in the morning. Thank you Elle for the Paleo Thyroid Solu-tion; you are my "Thyroid Hero!"

MORGAN—AUGUST 2015 *(On .75 grains of NDT)*

TEST	RESULT	RANGE
TSH	0.018	(0.450–4.500)
Free T4	0.97	(0.82–1.77)
Free T3	3.1	(2.0–4.4)

A year later, on .75 grains of NDT. My TSH is more supressed, and my Free T3 moved up. I am feeling good, yet I plan on experimenting with my doctor by moving from .75 grains to 1 grain of NDT. I am back to my normal weight though and feel pretty darn good!

Cara's Story

When I look back on my life, I realize that I had hypothyroid symptoms for most of it. One I can recall clearly is that I was always cold. It could be 95°F outside and I would be freezing.

I was diagnosed with hypothyroidism about twelve years ago, when I had my second miscarriage in a year. My OB referred me to a well-known endocrinologist in Los Angeles, who immediately ran tests, diagnosed hypothyroidism, and without blinking an eye, started me on Synthroid (levothyroxine).

For about eight years I was diligent about taking my Synthroid pill every morning and getting my blood work done every three months. During that time I felt terrible. I was experiencing a wide range of symptoms, including fatigue (even though I was getting enough rest); weight gain (even though I was exercising like a pro athlete and eating healthfully); hair loss, cracked/dry skin; allergies (to everything); miscarriages; acne; heavy bleeding during my periods and long periods (more than seven days); and brain fog and emotional highs and lows.

Every time I would go in to see the endocrinologist, he would tell me my blood work was good and fell within the normal range. He would update my prescription and send me on my way. Several times I complained about having no energy and gaining weight. He told me I was probably just eating too much. (I was training for a marathon at the time.) When I asked about other options for medication, he just said Synthroid was the only option. Nothing else worked for hypothyroidism. I trusted that my endocrinologist new what he was talking about.

One day I was due to have my blood work done, and I was just too exhausted to drive the 5 miles to my endocrinologist, so I made an appointment with my internist, who is located less than a mile from my house. She did all my blood work and when she went over the results with me, she said "Your thyroid results are low, and did you know you have Hashimoto's? I'm not sure why your endocrinologist has you on Synthroid…it doesn't work well for people with Hashimoto's." This doctor appointment changed my life. My internist prescribed a new compounded medication for me (T4/T3 combination) that day, and I started taking it immediately.

After that appointment I went home and curled up on my bed and cried for the rest of the day. I was so angry and depressed that my endocrinologist never tested my thyroid antibodies to find out whether or not I had Hashimoto's. How could he have misdiagnosed me and mistreated me for *eight years*? I was beside myself, because he not only ignored and dismissed all of my complaints, but also he made me feel as if I were a crazy person and a hypochondriac.

A week later I went back to my internist and she took some intensive blood tests to check all my vitamin and mineral levels. When we went over the results of those tests, she said to me, "If you were not sitting in front of me right now I would have concluded (based on the results of your tests) that you were a person who is going through chemotherapy. Your immune system is severely compromised."

We immediately started a vitamin/mineral protocol to get my immune system back into shape. I am happy to say that after a year of supplementation, along with the new medication, my thyroid and immune system started to work properly again.

For eight years I suffered with massive hypothyroid symptoms and didn't even realize it until my new compounded T4/T3 medication kicked in and I started feeling better—in fact, I felt amazing! All of my hypothyroid symptoms went away. I was losing weight; feeling smarter/more focused (my brain fog vanished!); started having shorter and lighter menstrual periods; free of all allergies (this was huge!); energetic and enthusiastic; and happy!

Now I go in and get my blood work done every six months. My doctor adjusts my medication, depending on my test results combined with how I feel. If I am having any hypothyroid symptoms, my doctor listens to me and adjusts my medication accordingly. I love that she doesn't just rely on test results and isn't afraid of a Free T3 that is toward the top or at the very top of the range.

I am currently on compounded thyroid hormone replacement equivalent to 4 grains of NDT. Even though my thyroid hormone replacement is optimized, I continue to take supplements to support T4 to T3 conversion and optimal thyroid hormone metabolism/adrenal health. I am diligent about taking selenium, vitamin D, vitamin B-complex, fish oil, and a probiotic.

After many years on compounded T4/T3, I decided to adopt a paleo/primal lifestyle. Elle had gone primal a couple of years prior, but she didn't try to convince me to change my diet and exercise lifestyle because she thought I would be the last person in the world who would ever be open to eliminating grains from my diet. That is, until Elle spoke with Dr. Gary Foresman about Hashimoto's. Very concerned for me, Elle immediately called me and explained the connection between grains and Hashimoto's antibody levels and what that meant for my long-term health. I was unaware that it was even possible to consciously lower my levels of thyroid antibodies, nor did I know that lower levels were better than higher levels. I assumed, like many (and my uninformed doctor!), that because I had Hashimoto's I would always see the presence of antibodies on my blood tests and that the fluctuations were random and uncontrollable. I was also unaware that higher levels of antibodies are detrimental to my long-term health and could potentially ignite other autoimmune disorders and other health issues.

Since I adopted a paleo eating strategy and lifestyle (including significantly reducing my high-intensity tennis workouts from three to four days a week down to about one day a week), my Hashimoto's thyroid antibodies have decreased significantly. Before going paleo, my TPO antibodies were over 200 and after six months of adopting a paleo lifestyle (with a few cheat meals), my antibodies dropped down to 70. As of June 2016, my TPO antibodies are the lowest I have ever seen them...down to 25! Having the lowest level of thyroid antibodies is my new goal. Even though weight loss wasn't a conscious goal, everyone in my life has noticed a major difference in my body. I have slimmed down even more and any inflammation/bloat that I had disappeared. The biggest change I've noticed since going paleo and becoming fat adapted, is that I eat a lot less food overall. My body is more efficient and I no longer have the blood sugar highs and lows that I used to. The cranky monster that would come out when I started getting hungry no longer exists!

Because I am the cook in the house, my husband accidentally (or by default) transitioned to the paleo lifestyle with me. At first he expressed some resistance, because he is a creature of habit and believes that every meal should have protein, salad or vegetable, and some sort of carbohydrate like bread or pasta. There were definitely some grumbles at the dinner table when I first eliminated grains from our meals. Soon enough, he actually realized that he was benefitting from the paleo lifestyle too. He no longer had arthritis pain, he lost weight, he went longer in between meals, and he had a lot more energy. My husband has come a long way from being a reluctant convert.

Of course I am human, so yes, I do cheat every once in a while! I have no guilt about taking on a slice of pizza or a bowl of pasta every now and then. That said, it definitely comes with a price to pay. When I do cheat with something containing grains, I get stuffy and feel bloated the next day. I also wake up hungry and feel stiffness in my body. I have noticed after a solid year of going paleo that I rarely crave sugar. Being paleo has made big a difference in my life. I feel so much better, and I feel so much freedom around food because I am not always thinking about my next meal.

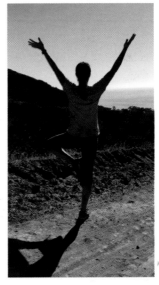

What I have learned through my Hashimoto's journey is that it is very important to get second and third opinions, follow your intuition/gut, ask questions, learn about your health issue, listen to your body, and don't let anyone make you feel bad about yourself. Oh, and *go paleo*!

I am so grateful for Elle and the Paleo Thyroid Solution, because without it I would have never known about grains negatively affecting my antibody levels—and that alone is saving my life! I am also grateful to have gotten rid of my sweet tooth and constant hunger; I feel

Cara - January 2016

free from an obsession I didn't realize I even had—until it went away! Living a paleo/primal lifestyle has changed my life and health in amazing ways, and I won't go back to being a sugar-burning grain-eater ever again!

ELLE ON CARA'S BLOOD WORK

Cara's blood results have consistently looked the same. Aside from minor adjustments in medication over the years, she mostly does well on compounded thyroid hormone combination T4/T3 (1 pill = 76 mcg of T4 and 18 mcg of T3). Since she takes one pill twice a day, Cara's dose is the equivalent of taking 4 grains of NDT per day (each grain or 60 mg of NDT = 38 mcg of T4 and 9 mcg of T3). Cara takes her thyroid medication once after waking in the morning and once in the afternoon at 4:00 p.m.

CARA—JUNE 2013 *(Optimized on thyroid hormone replacement)*

TEST	RESULT	RANGE	NOTES
Free T3	4.6	(2.3–4.2)	over range
Free T4	1.4	(0.8–1.8)	mid-range
TSH	0.01	(0.40–4.50)	"suppressed"

CARA—SEPTEMBER 2014 *(Optimized on thyroid hormone replacement)*

TEST	RESULT	RANGE	NOTES
Free T3	3.9	(2.3–4.2)	over mid-range and toward top of range
Free T4	1.2	(0.8–1.8)	almost at mid-range
TSH	0.01	(0.40–4.50)	"suppressed"

Cara is slim, very healthy, vibrant, and feels great! You'll notice Cara's TSH is suppressed—a common end-result of being optimized on a T4/T3 combination. You'll also notice that Cara's Free T3 is a few points *over* the range on the first panel. This normally does not alarm her doctor because Cara's Free T4 is mid-range and not high in the range, which could indicate hyperthyroidism or a T4 to T3 conversion issue. On the second test panel above, you'll notice Cara's Free T3 is pretty much at the top of the range, just a few points under. Her Free T4 is a couple of points below the mid-range. Cara's above labs reflect her seasonal medication adjustment (slightly higher dosage in winter, and slightly lower in summer).

Cara felt no difference in her health between the above two blood panels, but her doctor lowered her thyroid hormone dosage slightly after the June 2013 test results, probably after seeing Cara's Free T3 over the range and factoring in the time of year, summer. Did Cara *need* to have her medication decreased after the first panel? Probably not; having a Free T3 over the range is not harmful, if the patient requires it and experiences no overstimulation/hyperthyroid symptoms.

Those labs were fine *for Cara*, and even though she had no overstimulation symptoms of too much T3, her doctor was being conservative. Cara has done very well on both hormone dosage adjustments, but her doctor was probably taking a conservative approach by slightly decreasing Cara's prescription last June at the onset of summer. And if Cara feels great with her Free T3 at the *top* of the range and she also feels great with her Free T3 a few points *over* the range, then between those two Free T3 values is where Cara needs to "metabolically hang out."

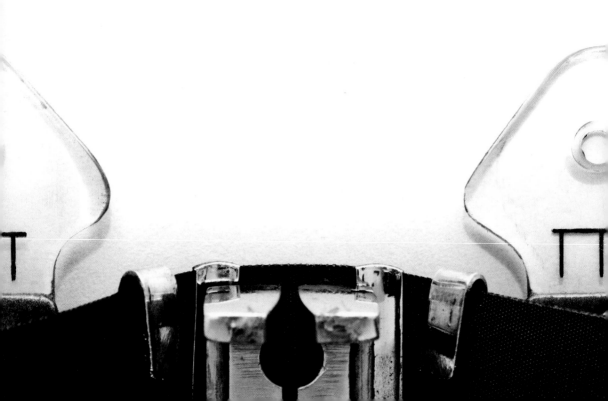
Don't Give Up!

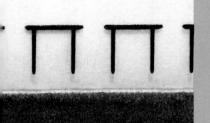

Conclusion

You may encounter many defeats,
but you must not be defeated.
In fact, it may be necessary to
encounter the defeats, so you can know
who you are, what you can rise from,
how you can still come out of it.

— Maya Angelou

Don't let anyone (not even yourself) convince you that you will always have weight issues, gynecological issues, or any other ailment in life, just because you have hypothyroidism. It simply isn't true. And more importantly, don't ever give up on yourself! When I was extremely hypothyroid, sick, bloated, and depressed, a family member said to me (actually they *screamed* at me), after they thought I had attended an excessive number of doctors' appointments, "At some point you're going to have to listen to one of these doctors!" Guess what? No, I didn't *have* to, and I am so grateful that I didn't take that family member's advice and listen to *any* of those doctors. I would have never gotten better; I would have gotten sicker.

I kept searching until I found the solution, and ultimately, I also found the right doctor. You must ask yourself, "How badly do I want to live a great life, with a healthy body and brain?" I wanted it very badly, and thankfully my burning desire led me down a path to the ultimate opportunity: being able to share my thyroid journey with you in this book and hopefully help change your life as I changed my own.

Believe in yourself. Learn to love yourself. Just know that anything you are struggling with thyroid or body-wise is temporary and fixable. Perseverance prevails. You *will* prevail if you set your mind to it and want it badly enough.

I have only one request of you, dear reader: When you achieve success with your thyroid health and overall health, pass it on and pay it forward by helping others stay off the wrong path. Hypothyroidism affects over 200 million people worldwide; you are bound to run into a few of them.

In-Depth Commentary from

Gary E. Foresman, MD

Founder and director of Middle Path Medicine, Gary E. Foresman, MD, has over twenty-five years of experience in the clinical practice of Internal/Integrative Medicine. Dr. Foresman is the only internist on the Central Coast with extensive research training during medical school as part of the then Junior Honors Medical Program. He ranked among the top in the nation on his Internal Medicine Board Exams. He has the best and most comprehensive internal medicine training to be found, including serving as a clinical professor who has trained other physicians at a university medical center.

In 1994, when he moved to the Central Coast to raise his family and open a private practice, he quickly became dissatisfied with the inability of established Western medical treatments to effectively treat many of his patients. Determined to help his patients, he began investigating alternative therapies and has expanded his training in many systems of healing, not just Ayurveda,

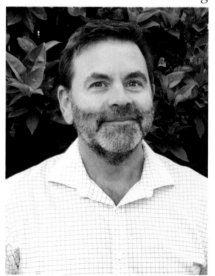

Gary E. Foresman
www.MiddlePathMedicine.com

meditation, stress management, and massage, but also botanical, ortho-molecular, and functional medicine systems. His precise, scientific mind combined with a holistic integrative perspective makes him not only the best diagnostician, but also the most skilled at therapeutically synthesizing the finest healing modalities for each individual.

Dr. Foresman has a variety of hobbies, including growing a vegetable garden, raising egg-laying hens, and tending to his household of four-legged friends.

Education

- 1984 University of Florida, Bachelor's Degree in Biological & Medical Sciences
- Member of Junior Honors Medical Program (accelerates path through medical school), Phi Beta Kappa Scholar
- 1987 University of Florida, Medical Doctor
- 1988 University of California Irvine, Internal Medicine Internship
- 1990 Internal Medicine Residency
- 1991 Primary Care Internal Medicine Fellowship
- 2010 Integrative Oncology Fellowship
- 2011 American Academy of Anti-Aging Medicine, Functional, Anti-Aging, and Regenerative Medicine Fellowship

Certificates and License

- 1988–Present California License to Practice Medicine
- 1990 American Board of Internal Medicine Diplomate
- 1994 Certified Instructor in Ayurveda and Primordial Sound Meditation, Chopra Center
- 1999 Certified Massage Therapist
- 2010 Fellow in Integrative Cancer Therapies
- 2011 American Academy of Anti-Aging Medicine Board Diplomate of Functional, Anti-Aging and Regenerative Medicine

Elle: In the twenty-five years you've practiced medicine, have you seen an increase or decrease in hypothyroidism?

Dr. Foresman: Unequivocally an *increase*, and the data out there supports that considerably. There is a significant trend, whether you look at blood studies, thyroid antibody studies, and even some of the autopsy studies. They all show unequivocally that hypothyroidism is on an upward trend, especially autoimmune thyroid diseases like Hashimoto's. At this point, testing my patients for thyroid antibodies is almost a regular screening process.

Elle: As for the significant increase in autoimmune thyroid diseases like Hashimoto's, what is your opinion on why there might be such a significant increase?

Dr. Foresman: So many factors. But let's look at the 1980s low-fat/high-carb diet craze, which led to an explosion of processed foods in general, which led to the obese-ification of America, and that led to a massive increase in metabolic syndrome disorders. There is a strong link between diabetes, metabolic syndrome, and thyroid disease.

Elle: Hypothyroid patients are more susceptible to getting diabetes, and vice versa, right?

Dr. Foresman: Right.

Elle: That makes perfect sense to me, because even if someone resolves their hypothyroidism naturally or through thyroid hormone replacement, they might still be *insulin resistant* from when they *were* hypothyroid—which happened to me. If that person doesn't transition their body out of that insulin-resistant state (which is achieved by going paleo/primal), they might never lose the excess weight gained in the former hypothyroid state, and it could also lead to contracting a second metabolic disease like type 2 diabetes, right?

Dr. Foresman: Right.

Elle: Roughly what percentage of your patients have hypothyroidism?

Dr. Foresman: Treating hypothyroidism is a significant part of my practice. Primarily because so many people who have thyroid issues feel mistreated by their previous doctors, so they seek out an integrative doctor like myself. A lot of people who come to me with thyroid issues have not done well on T4-only prescriptions, and often their previous doctors refused to order blood tests requested by the patient, or the doctor just failed to order the correct blood tests in general. I would say about 10%–20% of my practice is comprised of patients with thyroid issues.

Elle: In your experience, are there underlying themes present in people with hypothyroidism?

Dr. Foresman: Adrenal problems and iron deficiency concurrent with thyroid problems are the most associated.

Elle: I have a friend with hypothyroidism, who asked her doctor if there were any other medication options for her thyroid problem, and the endocrinologist replied, "No. Synthroid is the only medication for what you have." She was on Synthroid for many years and then started to gain weight and feel awful. Her endocrinologist kept telling her that she was probably eating too much and accused her of having a closet eating problem. She finally saw another doctor, who tested her for Hashimoto's and ultimately prescribed my friend compounded T4/T3, which she has been thriving on for over seven years now.

Why do most endocrinologists strictly use T4-only for treating hypothyroidism? Also, why have I heard from over forty endocrinologists, when I asked them if they prescribed NDT, "NDT is for pigs, not humans." Why would an endocrinologist say that about a substance that millions of people have thrived on and that has been around fifty-plus years before Synthroid was?

Dr. Foresman: It's part of the indoctrination. Being a doctor means to be indoctrinated into a way of treating people and it is truly an indoctrination. As you get more specialized in medicine, you are therefore more into it, more invested in believing in that way of being. And if you spend four years in medical school, another three years in residency, another two to three years in your endocrinology residencies and fellowships, the more you do that, the more indoctrinated you become into believing what you are indoctrinated in. It's not the teaching as much as the indoctrination. So a T4-only endocrinologist might be thinking, "Gee I couldn't have spent that much money and that much time and not be taught everything I needed to know. So since I wasn't taught about natural thyroid, Reverse T3, or compounding medication, it can't possibly be useful." It's a belief, a way of being.

Elle: Seems like a narrow minded, ego-based approach to medicine, which continues to cause harm to thyroid patients. Aside from that, it's faulty logic "I can't consider any other treatment options or tests because I was only taught to take these two tests in my medical training twenty years ago." Is this really happening? Are doctors actually reasoning that way?

Dr. Foresman: That's right, it's the idea of, "I can't consider anything else because I am so invested in this one view of thyroid health being true." So once a doctor has gotten to that point, they have the blinders on and they don't even look into the literature. And this is not just true for an endocrinologist. If you're a chemotherapy doctor, the only thing that exists in your treatment world is chemotherapy, and you cannot look at anything else because you have to believe in it, because you've been indoctrinated. The "chemo" in this case, is Synthroid (T4-only). It's the *only prescription* that doctors are supposed to use according to old-world conventional thyroid wisdom. Synthroid (T4-only) is considered a valid hormone replacement therapy because it does work in some people. But every good lie has some truth to it, which is for the good T4 to T3 converters, T4-only treatment is fine. It was *more fine* thirty years ago than it is now though.

Elle: Why is that? There are tons of patients out there who *were* doing well on T4-only but then had hypothyroid symptoms return and

T4-only stopped working. Those people went on NDT and began to thrive again. Why does this happen?

Dr. Foresman: I think it has to do with the metabolic shift that has happened in America. For example, we see a correlation between high CRP (C Reactive Protein) and high waist circumference, and also a correlation between high Reverse T3s and lower Free T3s. The metabolic shift in our country has made thyroid hormone metabolism so much more of an issue.

Elle: That's where eating and living a paleo lifestyle comes in and saves the day. I discuss paleo nutrition and its correlation with thyroid health and general wellness in this book.

Elle: Because you are an integrative medical doctor, a lot of people seek you out [because of their] complex health issues and/or because they are dissatisfied with previous doctors. What is it about these former doctors that drives a patient away?

Dr. Foresman: Mainly it's because the doctors refuse to take a test that the patient requested. To me, that is the greatest form of arrogance, because it probably means that they don't want to learn about that. And that is so disheartening to me because, you know, classically when you went to medical school, these were inquisitive, intelligent, people. If they didn't know about it, they would look into it.

Elle: On that note, I recently went to an endocrinologist with a hypothyroid patient who has been mistreated on T4-only treatment for fifteen to twenty years. She is overweight, miserable, depressed, and starting menopause. I asked the endocrinologist to test her Reverse T3 and Free T3. The endocrinologist said very patronizingly to me, "We don't test Reverse T3, that's old-school."

I responded, "It's not old-school because I just recovered from a severe Reverse T3 problem, so it's pretty *new-school* to me. Just please test this patient's Reverse T3 and Free T3."

Reluctantly, the endocrinologist agreed, "Fine, but I won't know how to evaluate the results."

I said, "Do you mean to tell me that you completely dismissed my Reverse T3 request as ridiculous, yet you claim that you don't even know how to evaluate a Reverse T3 test? Why would you *reject something* you know nothing about?"

"I am not going to be told how to practice medicine," she said.

I responded, "I am not telling you how to practice medicine, but I am telling you that your close-minded and outdated view of thyroid health is hurting patients. You are without a doubt hurting *this* patient." She was in shock that I even challenged her. She possessed the ultimate arrogance.

It is all too common that hypothyroid patients are belittled by patronizing doctors who practice ego-based medicine and reject the patient's symptoms and lab requests. Of course, it turns out that the patient did have a Reverse T3 problem, extremely low Free T3, and major adrenal dysfunction. This endocrinologist didn't even listen to my friend's complaints about her horrific symptoms. She didn't even look the patient in the eyes once during the entire visit. The endocrinologist just prescribed the patient *more* T4 at the end of our appointment. At that point I begged her to at the very least add 5 mcg of Cytomel (T3) to the patient's prescription. She reluctantly agreed. Since then, the patient has dropped 20 lbs pounds with some minor symptoms alleviated, but she is still under the care of this endocrinologist and not being treated properly for her Reverse T3 issue.

Dr. Foresman: That experience is very common. The saying goes, "You can't find a fever unless you take a temperature." So, you can't find these problems unless you measure them. So one of those indoctrinated endocrinologists who would say that Reverse T3 is never a problem, when is the last time you think they ordered a Reverse T3 test? Of course the answer is never, so that's why Reverse T3 is never a problem.

Elle: Are you saying that their philosophy is: *it's never a problem if you never test it?* That is beyond frustrating.

Dr. Foresman: That's right. For example, a doctor may not measure iron stores (ferritin), despite a female patient complaining of heavy periods. That doctor might have taken other blood tests showing that the patient is not "anemic" per se, but then the doctor doesn't see that the iron stores are inadequate.

Elle: And if ferritin levels are not adequate (~50–100 range) a couple of things can happen. One is that the patient will not be able to properly raise thyroid hormone doses without issues. And no matter how much T4-only or NDT someone is taking, if ferritin is low, whatever they are taking won't work well, and they will still fell hypothyroid, despite being on thyroid medication. A lot of doctors don't understand testing this "behind-the-scenes" component of ferritin. Essentially, a patient can keep complaining of hypothyroid symptoms—no matter how much thyroid hormone is given to them—but until they resolve the underlying causes of the medication not working (like iron and adrenals), they will never recover.

Dr. Foresman: Correct. See, doctors are not testing for *thyroid hormone metabolism.* And frankly, in today's world there are so many environmental toxic elements like grains, bromine, fluoride, and other chemicals that can affect thyroid hormone metabolism negatively. You must look for and test underlying causes and triggers of dysfunctional thyroid hormone metabolism.

Dr. Foresman: Let's go back to the T4-only prescribing doctor. The confusion for such an "indoctrinated doctor" is that they think, "If a patient's Free T4 is fine, then the patient is getting enough T4, and since T4 *has to be everything,* then why bother testing the Free T3 because Synthroid (T4-only) is all I can give the patient anyway?"

Elle: I get that, but if T4's "job and goal" is to convert into the biologically active T3, and adequate levels of T3 are what keep us all alive and well, it seems *logical* to me to test Free T3, *to test the stuff that matters*, right? Is it that doctors didn't learn that T3 was the biologically active hormone in medical school? I am not a doctor, but even based on the limited outdated information that doctors *did* learn, not testing Free T3 seems very unwise in my opinion. Why wouldn't doctors think to test the *most important hormone* to make sure that the T4 converted properly into adequate amounts of T3?

Dr. Foresman: They just don't consider it part of what they do. For many doctors, asking them to test the Free T3 is like asking a rabbi how many Hail Marys to do—it's just not a fair question from the get-go. Asking most doctors to test Free T3 or prescribe T3-only when they don't do it, it hits them exactly like the Hail Mary request hits the rabbi; it's akin to attacking the "religion" of the doctor.

Elle: I still don't get why doctors wouldn't even *think* to test for Free T3 though. If you know that T4 is supposed to convert into T3, why wouldn't anyone *think* to test Free T3? Even in the limited worldview of most doctors, it seems like a huge blunder. I know I am repeating myself here, but I still just don't understand why they wouldn't test the thing that matters most?

Dr. Foresman: Here's why: their training is such that *only T3 in the tissue matters*, and the Free T3 in the serum is not an accurate reflection of intracellular T3.

Elle: Ah, so doctors won't test the Free T3 because they think it is an *invalid* test to begin with? But they think testing Free T4 is *more* valid?

Dr. Foresman: They think Free T4 is more valid because T4 is more stable, and there is truth to that. Free T3 fluctuates much more than Free T4.

Elle: So you can have a "normal" looking Free T4 but have a very low, "unhealthy" Free T3, and that's the reason doctors should test the Free T3 *and* the Free T4?

Dr. Foresman: Doctors should absolutely test Free T3 along with Free T4. However, the reason most doctors aren't testing Free T3 (other than the indoctrination element) is that the "big lie" about not testing Free T3 is still *partially true*. The reason it is partially true is that there is a lot of instability in Free T3 relative to Free T4.

Elle: So then, if Free T4 is more stable, why do *you* test Free T3 and suggest that other doctors test for it?

Dr. Foresman: Because the Free T3 result actually correlates better with how people are feeling.

Elle: So even though you didn't learn about testing Free T3 in medical school, over time you realized how valid it was and started testing it?

Dr. Foresman: Absolutely. And if you look up studies, they are starting to measure it across the globe now.

Elle: Low levels of Free T3 are linked with depression, infertility, insulin resistance, and more.

Dr. Foresman: Turns out that the reason testing Free T3 wasn't ever "validated" is that doctors didn't believe in it; therefore, they didn't test Free T3 very often. As a result, there weren't many double-blind trials to prove anything about it. That's the way it goes in most of medicine: the primary driver of the research behind thyroid health is pharmaceutical companies. If the only incentive of a pharmaceutical company is to make sure Dr. John Doe is prescribing T4-only, the pharmaceutical company is going to immediately dis-incentivize any research that looks at contrasting theories regarding thyroid treatment.

Elle: Synthroid (T4-only) is the number one selling drug in America.

Dr. Foresman: You have to understand that pharmaceutical companies control the research going on at universities. If something was being researched (even in someone else's department at the university), and that research threatened the pharmaceutical company's products, the pharmaceutical company will threaten to take away big-time money from that other person's project. Look, if your research on another project threatens profits of the drug company, your research efforts will get scrubbed immediately. Drug companies are quite an influence.

Elle: Which reminds me of what happened when Synthroid was patented in the fifties. Desiccated thyroid was working well for patients for more than fifty years before Synthroid, but drug companies couldn't legally patent desiccated porcine thyroid gland (a T4/T3 combo), so they made synthetic T4 (which they *could* patent). Coincidentally and conveniently, right around the same time Synthroid appeared on the scene, propaganda against desiccated thyroid emerged, like articles claiming that desiccated was unstable and an inferior choice of thyroid treatment. To this day, doctors still say tell patients that desiccated is unstable and that it varies from one dosage to the next. Desiccated is perfectly stable, it is a USP standardized amount of T4 and T3 in each grain of desiccated thyroid. Why do doctors still tell patients that desiccated thyroid (NDT) is unstable?

Dr. Foresman: Desiccated (NDT) is *not* unstable. It is perfectly standardized, tested, and very reliable.

Elle: So, what's the problem then? Are these doctors just not "looking into it?"

Dr. Foresman: Exactly. I was taught the same thing, that desiccated thyroid is unstable and varies from one dose to the next.

Elle: That's what you were taught in medical school?

Dr. Foresman: We all were. So think about it: why would an indoctrinated doctor ever prescribe something so variable and unstable, right? And in their outdated, old-school thyroid worldview, one doesn't need T3, so why not just use T4 since T3 doesn't matter anyway. See how that goes?

Elle: I see how it goes, but I don't like what I see. Millions of people worldwide, including myself, have suffered immensely because of Big Pharma's influence combined with the narrow minds of doctors. I suffered greatly, undiagnosed for over a year because over twenty of these indoctrinated doctors solely tested my TSH to diagnose me, and not one of them tested my Free T3 or Free T4, which was *below the range* and at the *bottom of the range* respectively.

Elle: Have you ever had disagreements with other doctors regarding thyroid treatment, and if so, what were the arguments about?

Dr. Foresman: Yes. It has almost always been an endocrinologist who questions why I am ordering extra blood tests for the patient, and the endocrinologist tells me that I am misleading the patient. They take offense, because in their mind, they are supposed to be the "specialist," and here I am ordering more specialized tests that the specialist refused to order in the first place. They get offended.

Elle: It just keeps blowing my mind that one of the main reasons why so many hypothyroid patients have been kept sick and continually mistreated by their doctors boils down to *ego*. It seems to be all about ego and Big Pharma profits. Where are the patient's best interests in these scenarios?

Dr. Foresman: In their [other doctors'] minds, my ordering extra tests for a patient undermines them. Even though I am ordering the extra thyroid tests for the *patient*, the endocrinologist takes it as an offense to *them*. In my opinion, our job as doctors is to *learn*. Unfortunately, not every MD has that philosophy.

Elle: I am so glad *you* possess that philosophy; it's why I chose to interview you for the book. Are you open to learning something new about medicine from a patient?

Dr. Foresman: Absolutely. I am always open to reviewing literature and suggestions from a patient and researching a subject further if necessary.

Elle: I asked an endocrinologist recently where he wants to see his patients' Free T3 in the range.

The endocrinologist said, "It should always be in the middle of the range."

I responded, "What if a patient's Free T3 is in the middle of the range, but they still feel hypothyroid and sick, because for *them*, their body might require a higher Free T3?"

He said, "Nope. Free T3 should be in the middle of the range, period."

I said, "Look, it is *impossible* that everyone in the world feels healthy and great with their Free T3 in the middle of the range. The reason I know this for a fact is that I am one of those people, and I know many other hypothyroid patients for which the same applies. Following your logic, if you were my endocrinologist then, I would continue to remain very sick because of your philosophy on where the Free T3 needs to be in the range. So, where exactly are you getting this very rigid philosophy on Free T3?"

He replied, "I get it from the American Association of Clinical Endocrinologists."

Dr. Foresman: That is the type of rigid thinking that brings frustrated, hypothyroid patients to my office. Every single person in this world is different, and everyone's metabolism requirements are individual and unique to him or her. Sometimes doctors will only "treat the numbers," and we have to treat the *patient*.

Elle: Let's talk about reference ranges on blood labs. Can you give us a rundown on how these ranges were created and why these are not anything to be rigid about?

Dr. Foresman: The thyroid test reference ranges are based upon average populations and based upon people *not* taking any thyroid hormones at all.

Elle: Doctors need to compensate for that when looking at these ranges?

Dr. Foresman: Right. For example, what you will typically see from doctors is that when they start giving their patients thyroid hormones (especially desiccated, compounded T4/T3, or T3-only), the TSH becomes suppressed, and that completely freaks out most doctors.

Elle: It totally freaks them out; I've had several doctors tell me that a suppressed TSH would lead to heart disease. I discuss TSH suppression in the book and expose the myths behind why most doctors freak out if they see a patient's TSH is suppressed.

Elle: What are the worst cases of hypothyroidism that you've seen?

Dr. Foresman: The worst case scenarios are always the ones where the patient has had ongoing adrenal fatigue for twenty-plus years sometimes, and at some point along the way hypothyroidism showed up (and was being mistreated by their doctor), so when these patients (mostly women) go into menopause everything is gone. There are no ovarian hormones left to deal with the adrenal dysfunction; they are complete "train wrecks"—they can't get out of bed in the morning, they are getting divorces, etc. This triad of health issues causes unbearable symptoms and takes longer to treat.

Elle: How else has hypothyroidism affected your patients outside of physical symptoms?

Dr. Foresman: Relationships and marriages are often affected. I have had couples in here where you can feel the tension between them. The healthy person is wondering why their hypothyroid partner is "acting this way." When you correct the thyroid, energy levels come back, natural libido comes back, and then the intimacy comes back. A relationship can turn around so much after the hypothyroid patient is treated and optimized on hormone replacement (along with the other elements like adrenals, iron, etc.).

Elle: I had a variety of relationship issues come up for me when I was hypothyroid (and when I was hyperthyroid), which I share in the book. It made me very sad to recall those moments, because often the patient *also* has no idea why they are "acting this way" because so many of them go undiagnosed and/or their hypothyroidism is being mistreated by their doctors. So, the *person* not the *disease* gets blamed, and often the patient experiences rejection by their healthy partner or friends/family.

Dr. Foresman: If no one knows what is happening on the inside, how can abnormal behavior be explained to a spouse, right? Until the hypothyroid patient is properly diagnosed and treated adequately, relationship issues are likely to continue because the underlying causes of the abnormal behavior are not being addressed and corrected.

Elle: I have read that about 14% of people with hypothyroidism have Reverse T3 issues, and that it's on the rise. While I was on NDT I developed a Reverse T3 problem, which I corrected with T3-only hormone replacement. Why do you think there is an increase in Reverse T3 problems?

Dr. Foresman: Stress in our society (physical/mental), and poor diet. You can assess the degree of a person's severity of congestive heart failure by measuring Reverse T3–it's one of the best measures–it is a marker of severe mitochondrial dysfunction at the level of the heart. So, it's a good marker of disease activity. It's a non-specific marker for wellness. I read a study where it was a marker for hyperemesis gravidarum (vomiting during pregnancy). You can tell when a woman is really struggling with that because her Reverse T3 is going way up.

Elle: And that is happening as a natural protection mechanism in the body?

Dr. Foresman: Right. The theory is that the body thinks it is starving, so the body slows down metabolism, so you don't become hyper-metabolic. I'm not saying we have to treat Reverse T3 to treat vomiting during pregnancy, but if you treated the vomiting, then the Reverse T3 gets better. That's why in so many of our patients we have to make sure that we treat all of the underlying disorders, because a high Reverse T3 is a marker for chronic stress of some kind, whether that's physiologically as well as psychologically.

Elle: So you're saying that even if a patient came to you and was not fitting a hypothyroid profile nor complaining of hypo symptoms, but the patient was totally stressed out or exhibiting symptoms of something else, you would test Reverse T3 anyway?

Dr. Foresman: Absolutely. To me, it's one of my favorite non-specific markers of wellness and un-wellness. In hypo patients the most common thing I see are patients who saw their standard doctor and complained of hypo symptoms despite being on T4 already. Their doctor gives them more T4, which drives the metabolic machinery to a higher Reverse T3, and their Free T3 drops even further. So when they come to me, they have these especially low Free T3s, super high Reverse T3, a very high Free T4, and a suppressed TSH. Sometimes you can make people better by just cutting back their T4 and addressing underlying elements like adrenals, vitamin D, iron, etc.

Elle: And in my case, when lowering T4 and addressing underlying elements didn't work for resolving my Reverse T3 issue, I started T3-only treatment (and still take T3-only). You have a couple of patients on T3-only?

Dr. Foresman: Yes I do have a couple of patients that cannot tolerate T4 at all, and those patients are on T3-only, in slow-release form.

Elle: I know everyone's labs are different, but when the Free T4 is over the mid-range or high in the range, isn't that an indication there might be a Reverse T3 problem going on and they should test Reverse T3?

Dr. Foresman: Yes!

Elle: When I had a major Reverse T3 problem, my Free T4 was at the top of the range, my Free T3 was at the top of the range (which has been normal for me), and my TSH was suppressed. My doctor said, "Your thyroid labs look great." She didn't notice the high Free T4, in fact she said the Free T4 "looked great."

Dr. Foresman: That's a big problem actually. The most hypothyroid patients, symptomatically, are the people who tend to have the highest Free T4s, because they complain to their doctors of lingering symptoms and the doctors keep giving them more Synthroid (T4). And even if the doctor lets the patient's TSH get really low, they still aren't measuring all of the other important factors like Free T3 and Reverse T3.

Elle: So a patient with a very high Free T4 might not be converting the T4 into T3?

Dr. Foresman: Right, T4 is *not* converting into T3. So the more Synthroid the patient gets, the more hypothyroid they will become. So yes, a very high T4 is an indication that there could be a Reverse T3 issue. The entire subject of Reverse T3 problems in hypothyroid patients is similar to the subject of women being told they need more calcium for their bones. It's not that they need *more* calcium; it's really a *calcium distribution* issue, where calcium goes to the places you don't want it, and it doesn't go to the places you *do* want it, like your bones.

Elle: So giving that patient more T4 is the "calcium" here. Doctors keep giving patients more T4 and the patient never gets better because the T4 is not converting into T3. The T4 is converting into the biologically inactive Reverse T3. Similar to the calcium debate, the T4 has a *distribution* issue.

Dr. Foresman: It all boils down to *thyroid hormone metabolism*. It makes no sense to give a patient more and more T4 if it *was* and *is already* being converted into the wrong stuff.

Elle: So what I am gathering from this is that all doctors need to start testing for Reverse T3, not only because there is an increase in RT3 issues, and therefore a need to properly diagnose people, but also mainly because thyroid issues are more complex and harder to treat nowadays? It seems like whether it's due to crappy diets loaded with processed food, stress, environmental toxins, or the grain-based government food pyramid influencing food choices, hypothyroidism has grown in its complexity over the decades. Therefore, if you are a doctor who strictly treats patients with T4-only and tests only Free T4 and TSH, you need to get with the program because this thyroid business has gotten much more complex since they went to medical school, right?

Dr. Foresman: Yes, hypothyroidism *was* easier to treat back in the day. It was a less toxic, less stressful world, and people weren't super-sizing everything. I really think what has happened is that the natural history of hypothyroidism has changed significantly. Each year it is *not* getting better, so MDs need to start testing Reverse T3 and Free T3 and be open to using other prescriptions, such as desiccated, compounded T4/T3, and T3-only.

Elle: Hypothyroidism is solvable, and it is terribly disheartening to know that narrow minds and severe egos of doctors, combined with drug company profits, are the reasons so many people are still hypothyroid even though they are currently on thyroid medication! The fact that some patients remain hypothyroid for twenty years due to this mistreatment breaks my heart.

Dr. Foresman: It is disheartening, and a lot of those patients come to me as a result of that mistreatment.

Elle: When I diagnosed my Reverse T3 problem, I assessed it by calculating a ratio between Free T3 and Reverse T3 (blood tests were taken at the same time), and I was told that a ratio of 20 and higher is considered healthy. Someone could have a Reverse T3 "within range," but the ratio between Free T3 and RT3 could be way off, and then someone could miss the problem. Do you also calculate a ratio between the Free T3 and Reverse T3?

Dr. Foresman: Yes I do. The ratio value of 15 and above is usually okay in most people that I see, but 20 and higher is healthier.

Elle: I discuss Reverse T3 issues further in chapter 4 of the book.

Elle: Do you treat hypothyroid patients differently now than when you first started practicing medicine over twenty-five years ago. And if so, why?

Dr. Foresman: Heck yes! I graduated medical school in 1987, and at the time we only had a couple of thyroid tests to take, the prevalence wasn't there, and we just didn't know about these other types of thyroid tests that exist now. And the epidemiology has changed.

Elle: So then what were the changes that showed up along the way? How did it "dawn on you" to investigate further and learn more about the subject?

Dr. Foresman: Simply, it was listening to my patients. Patients on T4-only treatment kept coming to me complaining of not feeling good. At the time I was only testing T4 and TSH because that's all we were taught to measure back in medical school, so why would I go and test someone's T3 or Reverse T3 (which you couldn't even really measure at that point in time), right? My way of treating people changed because my thyroid patients were not doing well. Unfortunately, the mainstream idea has been that everyone can just go on Synthroid (T4-only) and be happy. If that's your worldview of hypothyroidism treatment as a doctor, then your unhappy patients will be seen as complainers who need a Valium.

Elle: Well, patients have actually been told exactly that. They have been told that they are imagining things or some doctors misdiagnose hypothyroid patients with depression or bipolar disorder and prescribe antidepressants and mood stabilizers. How did you know there was more to thyroid health than just prescribing T4-only?

Dr. Foresman: A lot of the changes have come because of my trainings in so many systems: functional medicine, orthomolecular medicine, and training at the American Academy of Anti-Aging Medicine—a whole variety of systems. And you start to look more and more, especially in functional medicine, to try and figure out what's going on. So the reason to measure thyroid antibodies is that we can actually do something about thyroid antibodies! The things we *can* do for thyroid antibodies are *mainly* through natural medicine techniques, that's why most doctors don't learn these things. Most doctors are "prescriptionists," so if there isn't a prescription for it, then why learn about it, there's no reason to learn this stuff.

Elle: So, seeing this recurring theme of people not doing well on T4-only treatment is what led you to delve further into the subject. What was that process like?

Dr. Foresman: I do have patients who feel great on T4-only and claim it has been a godsend for them, and the labs of those patients look great; so in that case I say "party on" with T4-only if it's working for you.

But with the patients who were not doing well on T4-only, my diagnostics changed. So, for example, when I started measuring Free T3 or seeing high Reverse T3 values (maybe five to ten years ago), I didn't even know what caused high Reverse T3 at the time. So I would research it, because now I've challenged myself to look into a new blood test to order, but I have to figure out what to do with the results. So after researching the causes of high Reverse T3, I realized what an important component of a person's thyroid hormone panel it is, and I also have a more comprehensive view of things. Furthermore, I still understand that I can't measure thyroid receptor insensitivity and so many other things. So, even with good thyroid tests and a more comprehensive panel, there still might be people out there that you know you are not treating perfectly, because you don't know what to measure. It's a level of complexity that most doctors don't want to get into and most people don't want to get into. So they don't, and patients suffer.

Elle: Let's say you have to put a patient on thyroid hormone replacement. Do you have a preferred "first order of business" with medicating?

Dr. Foresman: Through many years of experience, this is the way I do things: I give a full thyroid panel on everybody: Free T3, Free T4, TSH, Reverse T3, and *two* thyroid antibody tests, TPOAb and TgAb. Everyone is different, but for the most part, if the patient is really low in Free T4 with a high TSH, a low Reverse T3, relatively high Free T3 relative to their T4 (because their body is metabolically efficient), I will start them on Synthroid or T4-only, because it is easy and will probably work for that thyroid profile. I *do not* use generic forms of Synthroid (levothyroxine)—this is one of the few drugs that I do not substitute. I had so many cases of patients' prescriptions changing, blood levels would change; I had a few cases where liver enzymes were going off after patients switched from brand name to generic. The lowest Reverse T3s you would ever see would be in a person going into thyroid failure because their body is doing everything it can to get every scrap of T4 to convert into as much T3 as possible. As you pointed out before, you can live without T4, but you cannot live without T3. So, sometimes when you have really hypothyroid patients with very low Reverse T3s, it is a herculean metabolic effort for their body to maintain a T3 level. If you put them on T4 and their Reverse T3 goes up, but the Free T3 doesn't come up as well, and you don't get the symptom relief as expected, then I will use desiccated (T4/T3 combo), and I mostly use Nature-Throid, which is my preferred brand of desiccated, except some chemically sensitive patients do better on WP Thyroid

Elle: Do you use Armour Thyroid (a brand-name NDT)?

Dr. Foresman: I haven't used Armour since they had a lot of manufacturing issues years ago.

Elle: I heard about that and wondered if I might not have been a victim of that. I learned that Armour changed the *formulation of the fillers* in their pills, and it messed up a lot of patients because it wasn't working as well. Forest Pharmaceuticals, who makes Armour, never told anyone that they had changed the formulation, so they blindsided patients. Doctors were not happy. I remember hearing of people getting sicker. I used to take Armour, but that incident left a bad taste in my mouth. Do you use any other brands of NDT?

Dr. Foresman: For chemically sensitive patients, I use the desiccated WP Thyroid. For extremely sensitive patients, patients who can tell the difference in a 1 mcg change in medication, I use compounded T4/T3. When you're talking changes of 1 mcg increments, you can only achieve that by compounding.

Elle: Right, because every grain (one 60 mg pill) of desiccated thyroid has 38 mcg of T4 and 9 mcg of T3, and you can't separate those hormones from each other or add/subtract values to them with desiccated. With regard to treating Hashimoto's, I have heard the following myths: Hashimoto's patients should never take desiccated; Hashimoto's patients should always be on compounded T4/T3; and Hashimoto's patients should never take Synthroid. Are all of the medications for thyroid valid for treating Hashimoto's (T4-only, T4/T3 desiccated, T4/T3 compounded, T3-only)?

Dr. Foresman: Yes, all of the thyroid replacement hormone options are valid. I've been doing this a long time. The argument behind the theory against desiccated treatment for Hashimoto's is basically, "Well, it's porcine thyroid gland, and you might be giving them more antigen that will cause more of an antibody response." I have tested that again and again, and again. If a person does the right things, as you get to in this book—paleo lifestyle, vitamin D regulation, appropriate selenium, managing adrenals, etc.—it didn't matter if I gave them desiccated thyroid; it did not make their autoimmunity worse.

Elle: Let's talk about iodine. All too often, a hypothyroid patient, or anyone looking to optimize their thyroid, will search online and find that iodine deficiency can be a cause of hypothyroidism and that iodine stimulates the thyroid, so they run out and buy iodine. But it can actually screw up their thyroid and even make them hypothyroid when they were just looking to increase their metabolism! I fell prey to that, until I said to myself, "Maybe I should *test* myself first, before taking iodine." So I did, and I was fine; I stopped taking it.

Dr. Foresman: Despite Dr. David Brownstein's book on the subject, iodine has not been the thing in my practice. And yes, don't take it unless you need it. I have seen more problems with iodine supplements with my patients in terms of complaints and with iodine screwing up their thyroid. Not just the TSH—Brownstein makes the point that the TSH will naturally go up when you start iodine—I'm not talking about the TSH, I'm talking about not feeling well, problems with Free T3 and Free T4, and detox symptoms. I am guessing that he has a different patient population than I do; perhaps it's because we're in California and get enough iodine in our food. People ask me about it all the time. I am open to people trying it, but it can make you more hypothyroid. So I am adamant that we check in on it and take follow-up labs.

Elle: I don't understand why drug companies who manufacture and sell T3 (Liothyronine Sodium) wouldn't want to sell more if it. Pfizer's medical literature on their T3 drug called Cytomel states, "Cytomel (T3) tablets may be used in preference to levothyroxine (T4) when impairment of conversion of T4 to T3 is suspected." So even Pfizer knows there are other medication options for hypothyroid people! Why wouldn't Pfizer and other drug companies want to sell more T3? There is an increase in cases of impaired T4 to T3 conversion in our modern world, why wouldn't drug companies push research to prove what is already going on in the world: people take T4/T3 combos.

Dr. Foresman: Think about it: selling more T3 goes against every mainstream, outdated, and incorrect philosophy that *T3 doesn't matter*. So they are not going to push the thing that doesn't matter, right? If they pushed T3, they would actually have to reverse their entire thyroid worldview that T4 is the only things that matters.

Elle: How do you take patients' symptoms into account with dosing thyroid medication? For example, do you have patients whose thyroid blood labs are considered "high" or "dangerous" by the medical community (i.e., Free T3 at the top of the range or a little over), but for that individual, those higher levels are healthy and normal, for *them*? And even though their Free T3s are at the top of the range, the patients are not hyperthyroid just because their labs might look that way to doctors who have a narrow thyroid worldview?

Dr. Foresman: It actually happens all the time. You have to take your patients' symptoms into account—symptoms are our greatest teachers. Your question applies in either direction by the way, there are patients who have a higher Free T3 and are doing great, and if they go below that they feel hypothyroid. And there are rare situations where a patient's Free T3 value looks a little low, and so you give them more thyroid hormone, but they start to feel awful and hyperthyroid, so you lower back the dose. In that instance, those individuals' metabolism requirements were perfectly satisfied with a Free T3 below the mid-range and they continue to live a good life with those levels. It goes in both directions.

Elle: Getting back to the TSH being "suppressed," we are talking about a TSH lab result that usually looks something like 0.01 or 0.03 out of a range of 0.40–4.50. Having a 0.01 TSH value essentially means that *zero* signals are being sent from the pituitary to your thyroid gland, trying to wake it up to produce more thyroid hormones. The TSH is suppressed because the pituitary senses the blood has enough thyroid hormone, because the person is taking thyroid hormone replacement.

Dr. Foresman: Right.

Elle: I had an endocrinologist tell me that a suppressed TSH could lead to heart disease and osteoporosis. Aside from the indoctrination of doctors, why exactly do doctors get freaked out when they see a suppressed TSH? What is the false reasoning behind this fear?

Dr. Foresman: Studies from decades and decades ago indicated that a suppressed TSH might be an issue. What they used to do more than twenty-five years ago was give high doses of Synthroid (T4) to patients with the intention of suppressing their TSHs in order to shrink thyroid gland nodules. A very bad, outdated protocol that doctors no longer practice. At the time, they used such high doses of T4 that they were making some people chronically hyperthyroid and of course were seeing bone loss, arrhythmias, etc. The medical community stopped implementing that practice because of those outcomes. But unfortunately, as a result of that antiquated practice, there are still doctors who think that a suppressed TSH is dangerous to the patient.

Elle: Old, outdated, conventional medical wisdom. So basically, a doctor who is afraid of a suppressed TSH is synonymous with a person being afraid of saturated fat causing heart disease, because people only remember the old, incorrect, and flawed studies on saturated fat, and not the latest research.

Dr. Foresman: All of the studies in the last few decades indicate that TSH suppression has no association with some of those feared results, like osteoporosis. Interestingly enough, my patients with the lowest TSH values have the best bone density scores.

Elle: The correlation between thyroid treatment and suppressed TSH is that most patients who are optimized on a T4/T3 combo end up having a suppressed TSH, right? To clarify that, using thyroid hormone to suppress someone's TSH is not the *goal*, but it just ends up being the *result* of thyroid hormone optimization, right?

Dr. Foresman: In my practice and experience, most of the time that is true. I have had patients move to another state, and their new doctor refuses to prescribe desiccated or compounded. And as soon as the doctor sees a suppressed TSH, the doctor freaks out and lowers the patient's thyroid medication.

Elle: People are suffering *right now* because of a thirty-plus-year-old outdated treatment protocol, which the conclusions from have since been proven false?

Dr. Foresman: It's an antiquated belief system based upon decades-old history of using suppressive thyroid hormone to shrink thyroid nodules. As a result, doctors are *still* afraid of suppressing TSH, even though the literature has shown for decades now that you can suppress the TSH with no metabolic consequences whatsoever. A suppressed TSH does not lead to heart failure, it does not lead to arrhythmia, and it does not cause osteoporosis.

Elle: Good to know, because my TSH has been suppressed at about 0.01 for more than eight years now.

Dr. Foresman: And you're still alive.

Elle: With T4-only treatment, however, the patient will *not* have a suppressed TSH right? Only with T4/T3 combos and T3-only treatment is suppression normal?

Dr. Foresman: If you suppress a patient's TSH with T4-only, you would be mistreating them. That patient will either become *hyper*thyroid, or swing the other way and become *hypo*thyroid due to Reverse T3 issues. Testing the TSH is essentially non-essential in patients on

T4/T3 combo or T3-only treatment. If you give a patient T4-only, you really should be testing the TSH—you do not want to suppress the TSH too much, because either of the above two problems can happen.

Elle: Why is the TSH suppressed so easily by a T4/T3 combo and not as easily by T4-only?

Dr. Foresman: T3 is more potent, so it will suppress the TSH more than T4 will, because T4 is *slower and steadier* in terms of affecting TSH.

Elle: Is that why you only dose once a day with T4-only? Is morning best?

Dr. Foresman: Yes, on the once-a-day dosing. Dosing morning or night is fine, depending on the patient. The reason to give T4 at night is, for some reason you get better T4 to T3 conversion (possibly due to circadian hormone rhythms), and I have seen that in my practice. However, for the patients who like to eat late-night snacks, taking T4 at night is not a good idea, since you have to take Synthroid on an empty stomach. On the flip side, with desiccated, T4/T3 compounded, or T3-only, dosing twice or more is optimal.

Elle: Let me clarify that just a bit. With *slow-release* T3 you can dose twice a day and have that be optimal. If you take straight T3, as I do, a more optimal dosing schedule is—three to four times a day, because straight T3 reaches full saturation within four hours.

Dr. Foresman: Yes, T3 has a very short half-life. When I am using the T4/T3 combinations, dosing twice a day is optimal. Even with sustained-release T3-only, I dose twice a day.

Elle: Well, the thyroid gland doesn't pump out everything for the entire day in one single shot in the morning, so multi-dosing makes sense, particularly when you are taking something with T3 in it.

Dr. Foresman: T4 doesn't need to be dosed more than once a day because it develops a steady state over several days. So it doesn't make much sense to dose it more than once a day. However, with T3-only or a T4/T3 combo, you do need to dose more than once a day because T3 is so short-lived. There are some patients who do well taking a T4/T3 combo once a day, but multi-dosing is preferred when there is T3 in the medication.

Elle: Do you divide the medication equally between the two doses?

Dr. Foresman: No. Usually it's two to one. So if a patient were on 3 grains a day, they would take 2 grains in the morning and 1 grain in the afternoon.

Elle: If you have a hypothyroid patient that you needed to start taking desiccated thyroid, would you give them 1 grain as a *starting* dose?

Dr. Foresman: Usually, yes. However, I suggest that for the first three days the patient takes only half the pill (1/2 grain) and then goes up to 1 grain on the fourth day. I do that just to make sure there aren't any strange reactions, as some patients are chemically sensitive and could react to a "filler" in the pill. Just to be safe.

Elle: I think that's a good idea, sort of a "soft landing" into thyroid replacement.

Dr. Foresman: No reason not to take it slow for the first three days.

Elle: Figuring out what the optimal dose of thyroid hormone replacement is takes some time because of how the hormones are built up in the body. So many times, the biggest mistake doctors make is after giving a hypothyroid patient their first 1-grain dose of desiccated they are not retesting the patient soon enough, and then the patient starts to feel worse. When you start thyroid hormone replacement (particularly a T4/T3 combo), you are *dimming* the TSH signal, so you have to get that patient a dose increase in an appropriate amount of time, right?

Dr. Foresman: Depends on the patient and their symptoms, but usually we will measure the thyroid tests about four weeks after, or sooner if they are not doing well.

Elle: If a patient comes back after four weeks of being on 1 grain, and they are still not doing well, and it's clear that they need a dose increase, how do you raise desiccated from there? Do you raise by 1 grain or a 1/2 grain, or... ?

Dr. Foresman: I would probably not increase the prescription by more than 1/2 grain from there on out. Also, sometimes 1/4-grain dose increases can make all the difference for a patient. So usually I increase by either 1/4 or 1/2 grain about four weeks after the initial 1-grain starting dose (if called for). The first parameter is how the patient *feels*, which is more important to me than labs.

Elle: So, then as the patient moves toward reaching and maintaining their optimal dose of thyroid hormone replacement, do you check their lab work every four weeks until they are optimized?

Dr. Foresman: Usually. This is what I do: in the first year of treatment I like to give my thyroid patients a monthly standing order for thyroid blood tests, for an entire year. This way, they can go get tested anytime if they are feeling like their thyroid medication is off. Clearly, patients are not going to get tested every single month, but I give them the option of getting tested anytime. Then they send me the labs for evaluation.

Elle: I love that! You are allowing them to participate in their health.

Dr. Foresman: This is a participatory process. Frankly, no one should be better at treating your thyroid problem than *you*. Unfortunately, people don't often order their own blood tests and cannot write their own prescriptions. After a while, for the most part, the thyroid patient gets quite savvy about their health and they know when their thyroid meds are off. They know. Sometimes, it's a *seasonal* thing.

Elle: Interesting, I have heard that some thyroid patients need a little *more* thyroid medication in the winter, and a little *less* thyroid medication in the summer?

Dr. Foresman: Yes. That happens all the time. And besides more or less medication for people, in some cases the person starts multi-dosing in the winter and goes back to single-dosing around springtime. It's individual, and doctors need to be flexible to those factors as well. No one wants to take too much thyroid medication, it doesn't feel good. Thyroid hormones are not "drugs of abuse."

Elle: I personally, have experienced what it is like to be on too much thyroid medication (hyperthyroid). You can *feel* it, and it feels really bad: you feel too hot/warm/feverish, anxious, jittery, noticeably increased heart rate, aggressive and/or aggravated easily. I have always been a high-energy person, but *hyperthyroid energy* is not pleasant to experience and the people around you don't find it pleasant either.

Dr. Foresman: That's the whole point: thyroid medication is not a substance of abuse.

Elle: It's so refreshing that you allow your patients to have a standing order for thyroid tests, and that you are open to adjusting their thyroid medication based on symptoms as well. Some doctors don't even know what desiccated thyroid/NDT is, right?

Dr. Foresman: Right, some doctors don't even know that desiccated thyroid is an actual prescription; they think it's some over-the-counter glandular supplement or something. When you walk into a lion's den, you have to know what you're getting into. Again, most modern doctors are "prescriptionists," and you need to know what you're getting into when you seek one out for health assistance. Last week, I had a patient come into my office who had great cholesterol labs, yet her doctor put her on statins (cholesterol-lowering medication).

Elle: Did he put her on a statin because the doctor was unaware of the latest research and information on how to correctly evaluate cholesterol labs?

Dr. Foresman: Yes. That doctor was using outdated, flawed conventional wisdom to put a patient on a statin drug *who did not need to be on one.*

Elle: Ugh! Statin drugs have minimal impact on the most important heart disease risk factors and have numerous problematic side effects that can compromise health. I pick up that discussion in the chapter on paleo nutrition. On this cholesterol topic, so many hypothyroid patients are unnecessarily put on statin drugs because hypothyroidism *causes* cholesterol issues and the doctor missed the *cause* and went directly to prescribing statins as the *solution*. I, myself, had terrible cholesterol labs while I was suffering from hypothyroidism, and as soon as I got optimized on thyroid hormone replacement, my cholesterol labs went back to healthy.

Dr. Foresman: Hypercholesterolemia in any patient is a signal to test their thyroid.

Elle: What about blood pressure and thyroid, I know a lot of hypo patients have low blood pressure, but I know a few mistreated individuals on T4-only who have been given blood pressure medication for high blood pressure.

Dr. Foresman: I see more of a correlation between high blood pressure and insulin resistance, in fact, high blood pressure *is* insulin resistance most of the time.

Elle: Has anyone come to you with untreated hypothyroidism that had underlying causes like adrenal dysfunction and/or iron deficiency, and then their own thyroid bounced back and recovered once the underlying causes were treated?

Dr. Foresman: Yes. The biggest success has been with Hashimoto's patients, especially if you catch it early on. They have to eliminate grains from their diet and adopt a paleo lifestyle, and work on stress management. When they do those things successfully, they are not autoimmune anymore and the thyroid antibodies are not present. It's a much bigger issue than being a thyroid issue, it's an autoimmune disease. It's an inflammatory process within the body, so if you only correct thyroid hormone and you don't deal with the underlying inflammation, that person is still going to be at high risk for cancer, heart disease, and on and on.

Elle: So, even a Hashimoto's patient who is optimized on thyroid hormone replacement and is feeling good, they still need to adopt a paleo lifestyle so they do not create those antibodies?

Dr. Foresman: Right.

Elle: Can you clarify something for everyone? If Hashimoto's disease is the immune system attacking the thyroid gland, what exactly is the immune system attacking? Is it attacking the actual thyroid gland? Clearly the immune system isn't attacking the thyroid hormone replacement that the Hashimoto's patient is taking or else Hashimoto's patients probably couldn't stay alive.

Dr. Foresman: The T4/T3 that the patient is taking are *hormones.* In Hashimoto's, the immune system is attacking a *protein,* not a thyroid *hormone.* There are two classic antibodies, thyroid peroxidase (TPO) and thyroglobulin (Tg). It has been shown that long-term cancer risk is only associated with the Tg antibody. Some patients have only TPO antibodies and some have only Tg and some have both. These are inflammatory processes, even though they are listed under the umbrella of thyroid health. Different things can trigger those two types of thyroid antibodies.

Back to why being grain-free is so critical. I am certain that Hashimoto's is a heterogonous group of disorders where the trigger is different in each person. The only model we really have for autoimmune disease is celiac, where even though your body is attacking certain enzymes present in the intestinal tissues and across the body, once you take away the trigger (gluten), then your body stops attacking you, even though you're still there. So, can a person stop making thyroid antibodies, even though they still have a thyroid? Yes! Part of MD training says that once you are attacking your own thyroid you are just going to continue to attack it until it's gone. And that philosophy is not true. Nor is it true that your body has to keep attacking the gut enzymes with celiac because when you remove the trigger (gluten), it goes away. We don't exactly know what triggers Hashimoto's, except we know that gluten can mimic the thyroid tissue protein that the immune system likes to attack. What is the trigger? Grains play a role. It can be gluten in one person, or another form of gluten like corn gluten. Whatever the triggers are, they cause someone to be autoimmune and if you take the triggers away, the autoimmunity disappears.

Elle: Gluten and all grains can mimic that thyroid protein in the body and so Hashimoto's patients need to eliminate grains.

Dr. Foresman: Absolutely. I push a paleo lifestyle even harder for my Hashimoto's patients. Look, if there is evidence of autoimmunity and we know that grains are one of the potential triggers of that—and in my experience, one of the strongest triggers—you have to eliminate them. My patients who stay on the paleo path have the best responses in terms of thyroid antibodies. I see it all the time, thyroid antibodies go way down when a patient does really well with paleo; the antibodies will be at 1,000 and drop down to 100. After seeing the successful results, the patient often gets too proud of themselves, strays off the paleo path, and the next time they come in for blood work, their antibodies are up to 300.

Elle: So let me get this straight. If you have Hashimoto's, even if you are on thyroid medication and you are optimized and feeling great, you should still eliminate grains because you do *not* want to produce thyroid antibodies whether you feel the rise and fall of those antibodies or not?

Dr. Foresman: Absolutely.

Elle: And the reason that person doesn't want to create antibodies is that the presence of antibodies is linked with other health problems like cancer. What is it about antibodies that send a person down a path to cancer or other diseases?

Dr. Foresman: Inflammation. Autoimmunity leads to inflammatory responses in the body. Antibodies are inflammatory responses. Hashimoto's is an autoimmune disease. It's unequivocal that having thyroid antibodies, actually having Hashimoto's, increases your lifetime risk of breast cancer, colon cancer, and probably a whole host of other cancers because inflammation isn't good for the body. So we need to ask, what is inflaming this person. Grains are one of them. So is sugar. Any of my patients, whether dealing with cancer or Hashimoto's, it isn't just about the right combination of thyroid hormones or drugs, it's about diet and your mental/physical lifestyle. Symptoms can be our greatest teachers—health issues can be a big wake-up call for a lot of people.

Elle: So, are you just born with Hashimoto's? Or does an inflammation trigger happen and then Hashimoto's shows up?

Dr. Foresman: That is a theory. Here is the old-school reasoning: We used to blame autoimmunity on a virus. The thinking was that a virus came into the body and the virus looked like some piece of thyroid tissue and so the body generalized the attack and attacked it. Look, I am sure it happens sometimes, this molecular mimicry. But there are also triggers present in food, environmental toxins, etc. Right now there is so little research, because why would they bother looking at the causes of autoimmune disorders when all they are going to do anyway is just *treat* the disease, right?

Elle: Is there any evidence that T1, T2, and calcitonin are essential? I know these three things are present in NDT but they're not present in synthetic T4, compounded T4/T3, or T3. Is there any compelling evidence out there suggesting these components are essential to long-term thyroid health?

Dr. Foresman: I don't know because I haven't extensively researched it. I've gone through a lot of thyroid research, obviously. Have I seen anything that makes me feel like those three compounds are imperative in treatment? No. That being stated, I do not know that they are *not*. I'm going to have to put that down in the "I don't know" category. At this point, I'll have to say I don't think I'm going to find anything critically compelling there. And I do not know of any research pointing to those things being essential.

Elle: What about situations where things aren't exactly obvious. For example, it's not alarmingly clear the person is hypo. You know how people with normal thyroid function often seem to have a Free T3 around mid-range (usually 3.2). What if someone has hypo symptoms but their Free T3 is at 3.0 and a doctor might dismiss them? Have you had experience with patients like this, where 2 points below mid-range can manifest as hypo symptoms in someone who's not on treatment and never has been?

Dr. Foresman: The short answer of course is yes. This goes back to so many factors. Of course, you start off clinically, right? What are the symptoms of hypothyroidism? A lot of the symptoms are vague, and anybody can have them. Exhaustion, weight gain, constipation, and so on.

When we get these standard thyroid tests, even when we do more specific tests like what we have in terms of the Free T3 and Reverse T3. You start to see much more evidence of wow, something's a little bit off. The typical one, as you know, is if the Reverse T3 is high because of stress or dieting or any of the other underlying factors. The real reason a person like the one you described is feeling hypo can be that they need improvements in Reverse T3. As you know, the key goes back to the doctor having an index of suspicion.

Do we measure thyroid antibodies in everybody and at what age? The incidences of Hashimoto's is roughly 20% in women, 10% in men. Is that a high enough prevalence in the population where everybody over X age—whatever number you want to use, they're twenty-five, forty—should at least have some antibodies, especially if there's any family history of autoimmunity. As you know, in the overlaps with type 1 diabetes, celiac, and all the other forms of colitis—so much autoimmune disease out there—you could make an argument for screening thyroid antibodies in everybody over twenty-five, let's say. Because part of this, as you know, isn't just the thyroid hormones. They are having symptoms because of the autoimmunity. Autoimmunity itself is enough to cause symptoms, even if you're not a hypothyroid. You can have Hashimoto's antibodies and be inflamed and your interleukins are high, et cetera, et cetera. You feel achy, sore, tired. Your issue is truly your autoimmunity, even if it hasn't gotten to the point of hypothyroidism yet.

Here we have this super-complicated level of things where now, the person is symptomatic and they are autoimmune thyroid—and it's not even their thyroid levels that are causing it.

Elle: You're saying that antibodies might be present in obvious amounts to indicate something's wrong, but maybe the FT3 and FT4 look normal. Is that a situation that happens?

Dr. Foresman: That's exactly what I'm saying. I think it happens because early on, especially in our younger patients, that's the more typical scenario. You have your patient, let's say your typical fibromyalgia patient or chronic fatigue patient, and now of course there is a whole lot of things going on there, but sticking with the subject of thyroid, their autoimmunity is a huge part of their disease. They're getting hypothyroid symptoms and part of the reason is their pro-inflammatory state. I really think what we're seeing, when we're screening now (especially screening earlier on), is that we're finding autoimmunity. And of course as you know, this leads to our interventions nutritionally (paleo), stress-wise, and supplement-wise along with all those other things like iron levels and so on. Another classic example is a lot of these young women might be autoimmune thyroid but nobody measured their iron. They're really symptomatic because they're so iron deficient and they're just a little tweaky off on thyroid. "Tweaky" is a highly medical way of saying it, of course. It's their iron deficiency that you really needed to treat or their vitamin D deficiency, etc.

Elle: What about someone who's got appropriate iron and vitamin D levels and is optimized in all the things that are considered underlying causes of hypothyroidism—and their thyroid labs even look normal on paper… for example a Free T3 of 3.1 versus 3.2, just a point below mid-range (which would be considered normal by most doctors' standards). Could it be that Jane Doe needs to feel better at 3.2 or above for her *personally*, but a doctor would discount her needing thyroid help with the rationale, "Your Free T3 looks good, your thyroid is fine"? Could Free T3 labs that are off by just a couple of points manifest as hypo symptoms for someone?

Dr. Foresman: Absolutely they could, and this goes back to the baseline level thing. The most important things in life are the things you can't measure, but measure everything you can. Having these measurables in people, even if they're fine, which is great, if you see somebody who's twenty-five and they have no thyroid autoimmunity and they have perfect thyroid levels, etc., now we have a baseline for that patient. Let's say ten years later symptoms show up. At least we have a baselines for this person: Okay, his patient really does live well at a 3.5 Free T3. So let's say now the patient has dropped down to a 2.8 Free T3. Well, for a bunch of other patients a 2.8 might be great, but for this patient who dropped from 3.5, let's say, it's not great. I see patients so sensitive to 1 mcg level differences of T3.

Elle: I am similar. I actually have done so much blood testing and then matching it up to symptoms. My Free T3 labs will look very different from other people on NDT. It always be higher than someone on NDT because I have no T4 present to convert. I will feel really hypo with a Free T3 of 3.9 versus 4.4 or 4.6.

Dr. Foresman: Each person's reference range is going to be different. I have patients that if their T3 was toward your levels, they would have palpitations, anxiety, and feel horrible. That's why you have to individualize your therapy based not just on the blood result level, but based on how the person is doing. As you well know, TSH is becoming more and more useless as a test, especially with anybody on T3. TSH is becoming a useless test in this setting.

Elle: Okay, the thyroid itself, if you have normal thyroid function, dispenses about 80% T4 and about 20% T3. So let's just look at T4-only for a second. It doesn't make sense to me that T4-only treatment could be an optimal replacement method (even though it does work for some patients) because that's not how our normal thyroids work. In my opinion a T4/T3 combo is way more optimal and more aligned with mimicking how our bodies were naturally designed to work. So, why is T4-only still being used? Granted, I understand the easy T4-only dosing of "once a day," but do you see where I'm going with this? Our thyroids give us some T3 directly, it seems insane to not give at least some T3 along with T4. Our bodies don't completely rely on T4 conversion. T4-only treatment makes no sense to me whatsoever.

Dr. Foresman: I understand. I think you know a lot of the politics behind why T4-only treatment became the number one prescribed treatment in the medical community. First of all, T4-only treatment is easy (when it works), and it also goes back to the discussion we had previously about the doctor not wanting to be "wrong." MDs were all taught that if you removed the thyroid gland, you could take T4 and it would be the exact same thing as having a thyroid. You and I of course know that's not true, but I'm just saying this is the classic *party stance*: "Just give them T4. Your body converts T4 to T3 whenever it wants to, so you don't need any T3." That is more or less the Western medical approach to this conundrum you're talking about.

It gets back to complexity because as you know, it's not like when you take NDT once or twice a day. Well, if your natural thyroid, when it's putting out this 20% T3, it's doing it in small amounts throughout the day and modulating, measuring, and doing all kinds of wonderful things that we kind of negated as being important. My guess is, for people who are less sensitive, the microscopic refined control of T3 levels isn't so important, and so they can be fine with just a T4 replacement. However, there's a whole bunch of people who are very sensitive to their T3 fluctuations and subsequently speaking, they do very poorly with T4-only treatment.

And yes, inherently speaking, it is not bioidentical hormone thyroid replacement unless you are given both T4 and T3. That being said, you realize that Western doctors don't care about it being bioidentical, right?

Elle: Okay. There seems to be a little bit of confusion between thyroid hormone resistance and Reverse T3. I know Reverse T3 well, because I have unfortunately experienced it. There are underlying factors that can affect T4 to T3 conversion. What about thyroid hormone resistance: That's not really the same thing, or is it? Isn't thyroid hormone resistance either something you're born with, where there is something impaired on a base level from the get-go? Can you give me a snapshot of the difference between Reverse T3 and thyroid hormone resistance?

Dr. Foresman: Thyroid hormone resistance is a category that of course Reverse T3 is one subtype of, because you can have thyroid hormone resistance due to a high Reverse T3. If you talk about that and put that to the side, then you basically have the issue with the people who are resistant (again, this is Western perspective) to T4 because they are poor T4/T3 converters. This has to do with all the selenoproteins involved in the target issues. Then, you have another subgroup that have T3 receptor resistance. That's the genetic thing you're talking about.

Even the one involving the enzymes is partly genetic.

As time goes on we're going to find more and more genetic causes for especially T3 receptor sensitivity issues, and then we'll realize those people need higher and higher levels of T3. You might even be one of them yourself because you need higher levels. Subsequently speaking, some people do better with lower T3 levels because there are probably *exquisitely sensitive*. We have to look at the other side of the equation. Are there people who are exquisitely sensitive to T3 because their T3 receptors are so much more avidly holding onto T3? You have to guess that there are.

Elle: What was once an appropriate dose of T3 for me (with no overstimulation symptoms) eventually transitioned into *hyper*thyroidism for me, and I had to significantly reduce my T3 dosage. At some point over time, the sensitivity got better, and when I look back on it, that dose became hyper for me about six months after going paleo.

Dr. Foresman: The sensitivity improved probably because of correcting all of the underlying abnormalities, taking care of yourself, managing stress, blood glucose, exercise, getting fat adapted, etc. When we use other hormones like estrogens, progesterones, and so on, if you use too much of them, the body down-regulates. "Let's just use testosterone." If you give a high dose of testosterone, it will down-regulate the testosterone receptors and therefore become more resistant to testosterone. It's like insulin resistance.

It's just, if you oversaturate with any hormone, early on you get a beneficial effect. Then, over a course of time, your body is always going to correct to some other set point that it has for itself. We just have to be elegant in understanding that there are many types of thyroid hormone resistance. The ones that we see day in and day out primarily tend to involve the higher Reverse T3s and all of the underlying factors that cause that T4 to T3 conversion issue. The conversion issues. We look at those types of things. We obviously can only, I don't want to say guess, but we can take an educated guess that the people who are needing higher levels of T3 and/or T4 sometimes are just having thyroid hormone resistance. There's all kinds of research protocols going on, looking into who these people are. My guess is there's a ton. I think it's not just Hashimoto's. Decade by decade, all kinds of thyroid problems are going up.

Elle: With the increase in incidences of Reverse T3, I'm sure it stems from what we've talked about before in terms of stress, poor nutrition, low iron, all of these underlying causes. I want to ask you about nutritional stuff. I want to discuss selenium. At one point, selenium deficiency could actually cause a thyroid issue, right, because the T4 won't convert?

Dr. Foresman: I still consider selenium to be number one most important nutrient for the thyroid. It's silly to speak of it that way because we're always trying to be comprehensive about all nutrients. But if you have to, for whatever reason, just pick one, selenium I think is the most important. There's so much evidence out there now linking lower selenium levels with thyroid autoimmunity, thyroid cancer, etc. Selenoproteins are really primarily thyroid-related proteins. Low levels of selenium, probably related to processed food. The majority of my patients, if you correct the selenium, give them 200 mcg twice a day (I use the methyl selenocysteine form these days), you will find improvements in autoimmunity, and that's a sign that you're having improved thyroid hormone metabolism and less reactivity to the cell. Selenium I found to be a much more important nutrient than iodine when it comes to the thyroid. I think it seems to be a ringleader in terms of the iodinated proteins as well. As you correct selenoprotein synthesis with extra selenium, you have a self-regulation of your iodine status.

We don't need to be putting people on high doses of iodine because, once again, the research on iodine, if anything, indicates more Hashimoto's or more thyroid cancer when you use more iodine. But I think selenium, appropriately used, 200–400 mcg a day seems to be so important for decreasing Reverse T3, improving Free T3, improving energy levels, decreasing thyroid autoimmunity. Of course, it doesn't always work out. It's such an important nutrient. I don't think it can be overemphasized.

Elle: What about glutathione? I've known some people who did a mineral/vitamin test and who have Hashimoto's or thyroid problems and they saw a deficiency in glutathione. Can you speak on glutathione in general and how it's related to thyroid health in what you've seen?

Dr. Foresman: Again, this goes into a world of oxidative stress. What we see out there is this oxidative stress and antioxidant/oxidant metabolism, what is going on in the body, and is oxidant stress bad for us? Whether that's smoking or environmental toxins, the problem we get with glutathione is: what is the best thing to do? Do you give nutrients to support glutathione synthesis? Do you give people glutathione directly or are you trying to stimulate your body to make more glutathione? Most of the trials—I'm using antioxidants of any kind (including glutathione) in treating almost anything—have been woefully unsuccessful, probably because of the "too much, too little, too late" phenomenon.

When we document somebody really low in glutathione, they probably had years, or even decades, of issues going into it. Then, giving them glutathione will probably help them feel better in some way. Energy, they'll start to detox a little bit, a variety of things that glutathione can do. Are we going to see dramatic improvements in their quality of life long-term? I don't know. And the reason why I say I don't think so is that we still have to get them back to what caused them to have these low glutathione levels. And what are the lifestyle issues and all those things?

If I used glutathione, I would either do an IV or orally with a liposomal glutathione. I have found sick people who significantly benefit from it, usually from short-term symptom relief, especially energy, especially thyroid-type symptoms, but do I get a feeling that long-term I am really correcting something by giving them glutathione? No.

Elle: Regarding patients who feel the difference in a 1 mcg change in medication, I've seen situations where people are *almost* optimized on NDT (or T3), they're feeling good. Most, but not all of the hypo symptoms are gone, yet the labs look good. Even a 1/4 grain of NDT can make the difference, right? Have you seen something that small make the difference between hypo symptoms and, "Ah! I'm normal again!"

Dr. Foresman: The answer is yes. On that order, as you know, if a Western doctor heard us say that right now, they wouldn't believe us. The key has always been, are you willing to experiment with the patient, not just falling into some normal reference range—my patients taught me this. Before I realized it was possible, I had patients say in the past, "I just want to change my T3 by a microgram." Of course, in the back of my head, I was thinking, "Oh, gosh. It's another crazy one, this is probably not good."

Elle: It seems like a natural reaction, considering your training and knowledge at the time.

Dr. Foresman: One might say, "Hey, what's harmful about changing her prescription by a microgram?" The answer is *nothing*, or change it by a 1/4 grain. You see, the medical training all along has been that it's not going to make a difference.

Then you try it. Of course, sometimes, it doesn't make a difference but many times it does, and you think, is it a placebo effect? It's a real effect. Then the next part of it you go, "Who cares if it's a placebo effect if the patient *feels better*." It's one of those things where you couldn't see enough of a change on a lab test to prove what you did was right or wrong, so why wouldn't you let your patient dictate the prescription to some degree? That becomes the push or pull between the doctor and the patient sometimes. For the most part, as long as the person's feeling better. Of course, I've seen it make a difference. That's the beauty of it, in some sense it's allowing the patient to run the prescription, as long as it's within reason, of course.

Elle: And I assume that patient wasn't exhibiting any overstimulation/hyperthyroid symptoms, etc.

Dr. Foresman: Right. There's also going to be cases where (and every doctor has had this happen) the patient is going to start thinking, "Whatever, I'll take 5 grains of NDT one day and 1 grain of NDT the next," and they're going to be bouncing all over the place. That just doesn't make any sense obviously.

Very rarely do you see patients like that. They're almost always like you, where you say, "Gosh. I just feel like I need a little more, a little less. Let's compound it. Let's tweak it a little bit." In the end, when you're feeling better, is it because of a shift in the prescription? Almost 80% yes. Is it going to be 20% placebo? Yes. Now, it has the locus of control in the patient and you can never underestimate the importance of locus of control in your health care in terms of, "I'm in control, I feel better."

Elle: Okay, what does *locus of control* mean?

Dr. Foresman: The locus meaning the location of the control. Locus of control with a person. That's where we want it because, in general, as you know, that's the battle today in the Western world, there's so many things battling the Western physician in terms of having any power in their practice.

Now, just as a side note, it's these new ICD-10 codes. They're completely ridiculous. I'm just giving this as an example. With the reimbursements as part of the insurance companies, you have the ICD-10 codes, which are completely changing every code that we every used. The only intention they have is to put another barrier between us and our patients. Meaning, there's one other reason that our patients are going to be mad, because they won't get reimbursed because we didn't put the right code down. They have made them more specific and they're really trying to screw the patients. What happens is, there's less and less control in each doctor's life. Doctors are seeing thirty patients a day. They're going to have no idea what to do with all these codes and what the patients are going to get reimbursed.

At some level, I think the average doctor has lost some locus of control in their life, and that they want to feel like, "Hey, I'm the one writing these prescriptions, damn it!"

Elle: Ugh! So sad.

Dr. Foresman: It's a lot of influences getting between the patient and the doctor nowadays that are so much worse than they used to be twenty-five to thirty years ago, when I started all of this. How that's relevant right now: if you have that backlog where the doctor is busier than they've ever been, reimbursed worse than they've ever been—I'm talking about the primary care doctor having insurance nonsense going on. The doctor is fighting back and wanting to have some evidence of control in their life, too. It almost puts a little battle between the doctor and the patient. I'm not saying it's right. That's the background we have to understand with today's doctors, is that for the most part, they've put themselves so far into debt, so far behind the eight ball, that there seems to be a lot more judgments from the doctor to the patient. If they want to individualize a patient's treatment and go past their knowledge basis, first off, that is a threat to their knowledge. Then a doctor goes, "When I do a little shift in the prescription and it's not AMA based (American Medical Association), then why am I doing this, and am I putting myself at legal liability?" Seems like a lot of docs work this way. I'm currently training a physician assistant. It's crazy how much she was trained by other doctors to be afraid of lawsuits. Seriously.

Elle: And if that is the first order of business with doctor-training, that's pretty sad.

Dr. Foresman: It really is. I have to reemphasize, patient care, patient care. Do not do things being afraid of lawsuits, because whatever you're afraid of, you're going to have more of in your life.

Elle: True. A rarity among MDs, you actually understand the concept of "What you focus on, you get more of."

Dr. Foresman: Right, exactly.

Elle: Laird Hamilton (the most famous big-wave surfer in the world) was interviewed by Mark Sisson for a podcast. When Mark asked Laird how he prepares for the worst fall on the biggest wave of his life, Laird responded, "You know, I don't prepare for what I don't want to happen."

Dr. Foresman: That makes a lot of sense of course, but that's what I think we're seeing. I hope you understand, this does dovetail to what we're talking about, which is that there's a lot of behind-the-scenes influences that will dictate whether the doctor will say, "Hey! Let's try that different change of prescription," instead of thinking, "Wow! This is funky and odd," even if they have some judgments about it; this is the low standard of care. The doctor is thinking, "What is somebody else going to think?" It is fascinating to see.

Elle: Thank God you're training a new era of doctors!

Dr. Foresman: There is some loss of appreciation, I think, for someone like yourself, you've been through so many things with so many doctors. You always haven't been appreciated or listened to, and I think that's an understatement.

Elle: So true. It's insane to me that many endocrinologists and doctors just don't even believe in Reverse T3; they think it's inactive with no physiological effect. They don't believe it exists, like Santa Claus. Then, you're like, well, what the hell can a patient do if they've got a Reverse T3 problem that doesn't exist according to their doctor?

Dr. Foresman: Right, because you're actually stretching the doctor past their knowledge base. Whether you're talking about Reverse T3 or you're talking about a few micrograms change or using the NDT instead of T4, you're actually taking people past their comfort zone. Most people aren't good at that, doctor or otherwise.

Elle: True, true. I know we've talked about Reverse T3, but let's chat more. Obviously adrenals, iron, and stress are underlying causes (possibly even starvation or overexercising) for someone's T4 to not convert to T3. We already talked about how you access it by doing a ratio between the Free T3 and Reverse T3. How did you find out about this problem in your patients who were not responding to T4 or who were having trouble converting the T4 in their NDT prescription? How did you discover this conversion issue? Did they just never get better on a T4-containing prescription? At what point did you say, "Well, you know, we need to experiment maybe with T3-only for this particular patient?"

Dr. Foresman: Yes, it goes pretty much like you said. The longest time in my career, maybe ten or fifteen years in, I didn't measure Reverse T3. It wasn't just me, *nobody* was measuring it. I didn't measure it because I didn't know what the heck it was. Then, of course, you always have a patient who complains of still feeling hypo, despite the T3, T4, and TSH looking good (or in some cases it might look like they're getting too much). So, you say, "Gosh, you're probably depressed."

Elle: That's very, very common.

Dr. Foresman: Exactly, so the faulty reasoning at the time would say, "Start with T4-only and if that fails, go for the Prozac."

Elle: Let's just say we're talking old-school, before you knew about Reverse T3 and someone wasn't responding to T4. They claimed to feel hypo symptoms and there's that moment of, "Okay, well, we're going to give you an antidepressant." But then, that antidepressant never really works does it? At some point, the underlying problem is still going to persist. How long would that Prozac work before the patient is back in your office complaining, and you think, "You know, this is not depression. This might be something else." How did you gauge that?

Dr. Foresman: It all depends, because a lot of people actually do have depression; sometimes it really does help the person, and it's a part of their symptoms of course. The vast majority of times, however, the person would feel better, number one, because the act of doing something and making a change helps people feel better. A patient might think, "At least this doctor's listening to me, they gave me a medicine and this could be it. I could be depressed because I *feel* depressed." Then, there's a placebo effect that works just like giving them the medicine, know what I'm saying? But that will last for a three- to six-month period, which has been my experience in the majority of the patients—because [in those cases] it really wasn't depression to begin with.

Elle: What you're saying is that for three to six months the antidepressant might work, but then the depression comes back, and you realize, "Aha! This is not really depression. This might be thyroid."

Dr. Foresman: Pretty much. You know that the person probably doesn't feel so bad about feeling so bad. Most people who have any chronic condition feel bad about feeling bad, right? No matter what it is. If you give them a little something to boost some serotonin, or whatever you're doing, they probably feel a little bit better, which makes sense. That's why to the Western doctor, it seems like everybody needs an antidepressant, because most of the people we see day in and day out have something going on, usually chronic, and it makes them feel bad about feeling bad.

Now, look back to the obvious part of your question, which is, you know that the next step is, what truly taught me about thyroid was always my *patients*. The ones that came to me and said, "Hey, I feel better when I do Armour or Nature-Throid," and I said, "Listen. I'm happy. This is thyroid hormone. It's not what I always give but here, we'll start using it."

Over the course of time, you start to measure Free T3 and recognize that T3-containing meds work better than T4-only (levothyroxine). They work better on average of course, as you know. As we've talked about before, there's some people doing great on T4-only and you never mess with them because they feel so good. My experience is that percentage of patients is smaller and smaller over the years for a whole variety of reasons.

Elle: Are you saying that more and more people are really moving over to NDT and feeling better than when they were on T4-only?

Dr. Foresman: I'd say the *majority*, now. In the past, my experience was, "Hey, yeah, 30% to 40% of people really seem to be doing better on NDT." It's probably 80% now, if they let themselves try it. Because remember, that's the thing, they have to be willing to try something beyond standard medicine. There are a lot of patients out there who don't want to do anything beyond what their insurance might cover and so forth..

It's probably been . . . . I don't want to mislead you. I don't remember how long I've been measuring Reverse T3s. Eight to ten years maybe? Not sure. It's something in that area. Again, back then, there was very little research, but over a course of time, you saw it correlating. Of course, as you know, Reverse T3 and Free T3 change so much faster than standard T4 and standard TSH results. It became something like, "Hey! We can really play with this and this will change much faster. We won't do your TSH and T4 every few weeks but we can do a Reverse T3 and see if we're making progress and see if that correlates with how you're feeling." That was always the coolest thing for me, which is, "Hey, does this stuff actually seem to correlate fairly well in the real world?" So far, yes.

You know, the basic Western medical model is not going to change fast enough for a person's practice, meaning if I had to wait for Reverse T3 research to come around for me to change my practice, then I'm going to be a dinosaur of a doctor. I have to *practice* this. That's why it's called *practicing* medicine. Back in the day, when doctors had brains of their own, sorry, that sounds so...

Elle: I get that it sounds judgmental, but it's important to hear this from an MD. And it's also true. Like when you spoke earlier about being back in medical school and how students were excited to challenge themselves, research, and problem-solve.

Dr. Foresman: It's true. And now, they seem to be so caught up in needing a double-blind trial before they can do something that somebody else isn't doing.

This way of practicing medicine is safe and it makes my practice so much more fun, because I am learning. You know, you talk with a patient, and you don't tell them that you have experience that you don't have. You say, "Listen. I have some understanding about this. We're changing your thyroid a little bit. It's really important to communicate with me. Tell me how you're feeling. Let's measure these other things, see if they correlate with how you're doing." Over a course of time, you realize, "Wow! This correlates so well. I get the Reverse T3 down and I get the Free T3 up." The person feels better in any myriad of ways that thyroid can affect, which is basically anything. Each person feels different, and better in a different way. It's astounding.

Elle: Let's say you see a very severe Reverse T3 problem, the patient is severely hypo and they are a disaster. What's the shortest amount of time that you've seen where a patient like that has been able to heal and come back around and be able to normally convert T4 to T3 again?

Dr. Foresman: You can *see* it improve in weeks, seriously. *Weeks.* It's usually more like months, because it really depends on what's causing it [the Reverse T3 issue]. The easiest cases have been people who were taking some medication or another that I could stop, and that was part of it. Then we put them on selenium. They were probably extraordinarily selenium deficient to begin with, and three weeks later, they're feeling so much better and the labs are so much better. I've seen Reverse T3 in the 90s before, so...

Elle: That is high!

Dr. Foresman: No, it's *crazy high*! You ask the patient, "How are you even *moving*?"

Elle: Most aren't.

Dr. Foresman: Yep. They say, "I'm really not, doctor." Crazy Reverse T3s. Obviously people with the most extreme cases get the most extreme improvements, whereas with subtle differences, you get more subtle improvements. You can notice differences.

Of course, as you know, during that period, they are instructed by me to completely adopt a primal/paleo lifestyle. They work on stress. What's making them better? Is it stopping the medicine? Is it going on selenium? Is it correcting their vitamin D? Is it having some fish oils? Is it going primal? The answer is yes because you don't get levels like that unless there's a ton of that stuff going on. You've got to do an intervention. The multi-factoral approach usually gives the most dramatic results.

Elle: I read something where a person claimed that T4 was essential for healthy hair, brain, and other functions, but is there really any scientific evidence that T4 is more than just a prohormone? I've been on T3-only for over three years. I have great hair, great brain function, etc. Is there any evidence out there that says T4 is important aside from its prohormone job of converting to T3?

Dr. Foresman: It's funny, because I'm sure that person looked at studies that would conclude that. If all they ever did was look at T4, and when you put the person on T4, all those things got better, which of course would be true because T4 is an important prohormone. Is there any *proof* that you *need* T4, other than as a prohormone like you just talked about? I don't know any evidence, and again, you know this, you have to couch this in this response. It's like the docs who say, "Calcium supplementation improves bone density," but they just lie to you, and they don't tell you that it's *only if there's vitamin D that's a part of it*. So they say, "If you take calcium, it can improve your bone density," but they forgot to tell the real issue, which is that the vitamin D is doing the work. There are studies that say taking T4 will lead to these improvements, but they never even bother measuring T3.

Elle: Right, they're not even factoring in, it's a false premise of a study from the get-go.

Dr. Foresman: Exactly. Of course, you can look at studies that will support a viewpoint if you don't want to look at what's actually happening. T4's job is as a stable supply of T3 for the body. That is its job. In terms of percent of function that comes from T4, I'm guessing there's a percent of function that comes from T4 that your body can respond to, but you don't *need* T4, no. My preference is to have some T4 around just as a prohormone, especially if that person runs out of their T3 supply.

Elle: Going paleo and getting fat adapted. Obviously, we know that getting fat adapted and adopting a paleo/primal diet and lifestyle helps with blood glucose management, and we now realize that old health paradigm of eating every two to four hours and remaining in that sugar-burning cycle does not work.

Dr. Foresman: Correct.

Elle: It's hard to connect all the factors involved with living a paleo/primal life and how it optimizes cortisol, blood glucose, and how that is helpful as an underlying scenario for optimal thyroid hormone metabolism, whether you are on medication or not. Now, when I went paleo and really stayed with it for over six months, I had to reduce my T3 dosage. Of course, I noticed improvements everywhere else, but what is going on there? Do you see what I am asking?

Dr. Foresman: Yes. I think the insulin resistance state, which is a pro-inflammatory state, which is what people get into when there are living a sugar-burning lifestyle, leads to a form of thyroid hormone resistance because they're in a pro-inflammatory state, which is a *stress to the body*. You look at the people in my practice and you see this all the time. This is the tough thing to distinguish: I have a subset of people who, when they go primal, I think the reason they do so much better from a thyroid standpoint is their Hashimoto's antibodies drop, and they really were having primarily an autoimmune issue.

Elle: So the fastest successes happen with Hashimoto's antibodies, where they go primal, they cut out the grains and manage blood glucose via getting fat adapted, and then the antibodies go down and they don't have to go on thyroid hormone replacement, correct?

Dr. Foresman: Correct. It's an amazing success.

There's another group that has a different kind of success, they're having the sluggish thyroid kind of symptoms. You can tell their thyroid hormones are off but not entirely. They're *sluggish* but you see they have these insulin levels of 40 and their A1Cs are early-diabetic, etc. They do the paleo lifestyle (this is of course for the people who *actually* do it). They're getting better because they are cutting out the carbs, not just because they're just cutting out an immunogenic stimulation, meaning something like a gluten or a glutinoid, and they get better and better. They get out of this inflammatory state. All their thyroid hormones get better.

Now, I don't have any science to prove this. I'm just giving my anecdotal experience but they're getting better because they're becoming fat adapted, and so on. They're decreasing insulin resistance. We know with high insulin, so many inflammatory mediators in the body go up that we take the person out of pro-inflammatory state. Again, are they feeling better because their thyroid is better or because they're out of inflammation? The answer is obviously yes, right?

Elle: Right.

Dr. Foresman: It's such an important part of getting people out of this sugar/carb-burning, insulin-resistant state. They lower inflammation, and it takes them out of the state of chronic stress, which is what is causing the Reverse T3 to go up. The chronic stress to them is being in an inflamed state. Does that make sense?

Elle: It does. So, this is my personal experience, and maybe you also have experiences with patients that had this scenario: You've been hypothyroid for a while, you've been untreated, you got fat, you're miserable. You get on the thyroid hormone replacement. You're doing well. Your thyroid's great. You're feeling great, but you just can't lose that stubborn excess weight you gained when you were hypothyroid. So, hypothyroidism that has been undiagnosed or poorly managed for a long time can throw a patient into an insulin-resistant state. Can you tell us the mechanism by which that happens? Because I think people need to hear it from a doctor.

Dr. Foresman: Being chronically hypothyroid slows metabolism, right?

Elle: Very much so.

Dr. Foresman: As we all know, thyroid hormone plays a great role and is essentially the metabolic engine that drives ATP production and everything else. As your body's gotten used to a state of being essentially undernourished (while in a state of being overnourished by carb intake, which means you're not able to convert the carbs/glucose into energy but you're still resistant to the effects of insulin in terms of getting the glucose into the cell, driving the energy into actually being utilized). What has happened is that you are almost in a state of *cellular starvation* when you have super high levels of insulin. Your body can't get the sugar into the cells very well. There are some studies indicating that using the nutrients acetyl-L-carnitine and alpha-lipoic acid can help turn on our metabolic machinery.

What happens is that you now start to turn on and make energy. Obviously your body just wants to heal. If it doesn't have enough energy, it can't heal. By making these shifts, we've actually corrected a very basic underlying issue, which is *making energy*. Once your body makes energy, it will correct so many other problems, from inflammation to high Reverse T3 status, because it's not under a state of chronic stress. To me, it's about stress. It's not just psychological stress that affects people so much. It's the *carrying the extra weight on your body* that is actually a stress to your body. And that stress unfortunately activates things that further slow your metabolism, further drive up your Reverse T3, and causes you to be in a worse and worse state of health.

Elle: Can you explain why a hypo patient who is optimized on thyroid hormone and feeling great should also adopt a paleo lifestyle to avoid running into a problem later because of the sugar-burning cycle?

Dr. Foresman: Yes. There are two levels to that, as you know. Number one, if they have autoimmune thyroid, and it's related to grains and so on, they're going to get another autoimmune disease anyway if they don't treat the cause of their autoimmunity, which is going to take them down another state of disease.

Number two, yes, we're always ideological, getting good thyroid levels is awesome and everything. However, you will manifest an imbalance of carbohydrate intolerance in any number of ways. Your body will warn you with high blood pressure, sugar, or lipids, even arthritis, or whatever; if you don't correct this underlying problem (which is switching to more of a healthy fat, whole food–based approach to metabolism), you're going to develop a whole new set of diseases, even if your thyroid is fine.

Elle: If you're in a state of insulin resistance but you're not on thyroid hormone replacement, and your thyroid is maybe fine-ish, but you become insulin resistant because of dietary and lifestyle issues, can that lead to hypothyroidism?

Dr. Foresman: This would fall into the category of age-related phenomenon, which is one of the primary bases of aging is, as we know, inflammation and glycation. So, as blood sugar levels rise and insulin (these are obviously correlated, but not the same), you get dysfunction of whatever system you're dealing with. So, if we're getting a little older and our blood sugars are going a little higher, do we have more of a sluggish thyroid that goes along with that? Yes. Even if you're not auto-immune, yes. I see so many people who were put on thyroid forever ago because they were told they had a sluggish thyroid and sure enough, nobody measured their antibodies. Let's say you measure you're antibodies. They're negative. Then, why did they get a sluggish thyroid? It's usually their nutritional status or lack of exercise or stress, all the things we've talked about. But, can just being in a state of insulin resistance through abnormal glycation link to a more rapid aging, essentially of your thyroid system, along with the rest of you? It's all just about aging, it's just about predisposition coming out. Some part of us is always going to age a little faster than the rest of us. In one person when they're aging a little bit more, it's really they get worse joints because everybody in their family has problems with arthritis. The next group is just going to develop more thyroid dysfunction because that's what their predisposition is. It's just about the aging phenomenon accelerating more than one part of your body versus the other.

Elle: Let's talk about a person in their sugar-burning state, where they're eating every two, three hours. Let's say they're feeling fine and healthy. Can you explain how being in a sugar-burning state affects adrenals in a negative way?

Dr. Foresman: Chronic up and down in your blood sugar is like being in a recurring state of stress. As you increase sugar in the diet, your sugar levels rise. Then your body aggressively responds with insulin to lower the sugar levels. As you do these rapid sugar shifts, each time the sugar goes up, then your body counteracts: "Oh my gosh! There's a lot of sugar here," and it brings it down. Over a course of time, it will always lead to overshooting, and you'll become slightly hypoglycemic. Hypoglycemia is basically the same thing as being under a fight-or-flight stress. Each time you go up and down in these blood sugars, on the down side (as your blood sugar's dropping) your body's going into fight-or-flight response, even if you think you have a nirvanic existence, you're essentially stressing your body. It's like putting yourself into a horror movie constantly. Then your body responds: "Oh my gosh! Blood sugar's getting low. Let's throw out adrenaline, cortisol!" It starts to raise the blood sugar. Your blood sugar raises, and of course, usually that is the time when you're eating your doughnut or whatever. That further drives the blood sugar up along with your high cortisol, adrenaline, causing an even higher blood sugar spike. Then, *boom*! It goes down even faster, leading to the next need. You're essentially under a constant state of stress by being a sugar-burner and that is bad for adrenals.

Elle: Regarding hypoglycemia. I hear this objection to going paleo a lot. "I could never go paleo or primal because I have hypoglycemia. I have to eat every two to four hours." My opinion there is, well, you wouldn't be hypoglycemic if you went paleo and got fat adapted. It just seems like if you have hypoglycemia then it's imperative that you go primal and get fat adapted to correct it, because otherwise you're just going to be suffering every two to three hours and have to have food on you all the time. Eventually, that hypoglycemia won't ever get resolved by "feeding into" the carb-burning addiction that is hypoglycemia.

Dr. Foresman: Right. Here's a parallel, "Of course I need heroin every two to three hours because man, I feel like crap in between." It's the same thing. That makes sense to them. People become addicted to heroin; it doesn't make them *bad* people, obviously, but it's not, "Oh this is *just the way they are*, naturally heroin-addicted." People get addicted to the sugar-burning cycle. Of course they feel like they need to eat every two or three hours, because that is the disease state I'm pointing out to them. Yes, there's always turbulence and you know that's why people who have heavy carb-burning lifestyles have the most difficulty taking on primal diets, because there can be a lot of turbulence that first week or two, right?

Elle: Oh, I had major turbulence in the first two weeks of going primal. Some people have very little turbulence. But I was a serious sugar-burner and insulin resistant.

Dr. Foresman: Transitioning to a fat-burner is akin to the addiction withdrawal that a heroin addict would experience.

Elle: Heroin being glucose in this case. Totally.

Dr. Foresman: Exactly! It's the same basic problem. Once you get past the addiction, then you realize, "Wow! I don't need to eat every two or three hours. Nor did I really need heroin every two or three hours. It just felt that way because I was addicted."

Elle: Obviously I believe paleo/primal lifestyle is the best way to live, but it seems as though it's the best way to save your adrenals and manage your blood glucose.

Dr. Foresman: Right. Trust me, there are people who you have to bring on board slowly because they're so attached to this world where they're supposed to eat twenty-two servings of grains a day, or whatever the ridiculous food pyramid says.

Elle: I wouldn't be surprised if they raised it to twenty-two! The government pyramid currently says we should eat six to eleven servings a day, plus two to four servings of fruit, along with other detrimental nonsense.

Dr. Foresman: So, if you take these people away from "their truth," which they are almost biblically attached to, it's tough. You are essentially attacking a core belief system of theirs. You're not in reality, but to them you are. This is relevant. So, for the most part, you get these people past the belief side of things, that's why it's great to have Mark Sisson's book and others to recommend to my patients, because I can say, "Here. It's not just *me* saying this."

Then, once you get them past the fear—this is especially true from the vegan side of the coin; they are convinced that if you eat anything *animal*, you're just going to drop into a black hole of doom, you know?

Elle: Right, right. Two of the things we hear a lot are, "breakfast is the most important meal of the day," and "eat three meals a day." Being primal and fat adapted is a different ball game; it becomes, "you eat when you're hungry, period."

One of the things I hear from everybody is, "Oh my god, traveling is such a joy being fat adapted." It's astounding how long you can go without food and have sustained mental and physical energy on every level with no drops in blood glucose, sometimes for eight to ten hours, which I experienced recently. I ate a beef burger patty with an egg before a six-hour flight to Hawaii. Two hours at the airport, six hours on the flight, then I get there. By the time I got my luggage and arrived at my destination, it was about *nine hours with zero food* since that burger-egg combo, and I felt amazing, was not cranky and starving when I arrived. It was perfect. Granted, it most definitely wasn't a grass-fed beef patty or an egg from a pasture-raised chicken, but it worked. It sustained me. Everyone on the plane was eating crap, and some of them I had seen eating in the airport before the flight!

Dr. Foresman: What you're saying is so true. You have to understand. Remember, the fight-or-flight response. These people have been programmed for hour after hour, year after year. Every time they went through a fight-or-flight response where they were hypoglycemic, they ate crappy airline food and they felt better, right?

Elle: Sure.

Dr. Foresman: They did. Now, they reinforce. "Crappy airline food saved my life. Crackers saved my life. Cookies saved my life." Now, you're trying to take away their go-to "life-saver." That's the thing. It's a very powerful conditioning influence. They know that crackers could save their life. They don't realize that crackers are exacerbating the problem and making them essentially more of a sugar-burner. These people are slaves to what they think is their own *appetite*, but it's not even their appetite anymore. They are slaves to a metabolic dysfunction that they created for themselves.

Go back to this freedom while traveling thing. What you just actually said was, "I have freedom more or less because I'm not a slave to eating what somebody else tells me or anything else." That's one thing.

Elle: It would seem like a real cruel joke from the universe or the aliens that created us (whatever you believe), that humans would have to eat every two to three hours. We would be the only species, right, who would be forced into that nightmare, and it just doesn't make sense. I mean, obviously there's too many studies around it and evidence that our bodies were designed to burn fat as the primary fuel and our bodies were meant to go long periods of time without food as fat-adapted humans.

Dr. Foresman: Let's make it really clear to people—that's one of the things that I found wonderful—is that sense of freedom you have because you're not a slave to having to eat in a defined way. It makes a huge difference for people once they get there. That is, to me, a selling point for what you're talking about; it really is a sense of freedom to choose to eat when you want to. You don't *have* to eat. One of the founding principles of our culture is this ability to have freedom in our choices.

Most people don't realize how many different ways they enslave themselves, and this dietary pattern of having to *graze* all day, it's just a form of indentured servitude to a dysfunctional way of being. Now, going paleo and getting fat adapted is just one other step toward freedom for them. It's a huge, huge liberating influence in their lives.

Dr. Foresman: As we've already talked about, there's more and more stuff going out there in terms of the importance of T4 to T3 conversion and how our lifestyle plays such an important role in that. The average Western doctor is coming around to understand the importance of T3. What you're doing is so important in recognizing the importance of T3 in the world. And we're continuing to read about the importance of thyroid autoimmunity from a standpoint of long-term, I'm not just talking about thyroid cancer risk or breast cancer risk. Young women who have thyroid antibodies have a higher risk of having kids with autism spectrum disorder.

Elle: I didn't know that.

Dr. Foresman: You and I both know autoimmune thyroid disease isn't even a thyroid disease. It's an *autoimmune* disease that affects the thyroid. The mystifying thing to me is how doctors forget that this is primarily a disease of immune dysfunction, and you have to ask what's causing the immune dysfunction. We've got to get the primary question back to this immune dysfunction issue; it's obviously a little bit more complicated. Of course we need to correct for thyroid. If a doctor doesn't pay attention and try to help reverse your autoimmunity, you are at such risk for other autoimmune diseases or having kids with autism spectrum disorders to having long-term risks of heart attacks and cancers.

I'm not trying to scare people, but this is an important thing, and it comes back around to the paleo lifestyle. *The paleo lifestyle is the key part of the cure*, if you will, in terms of really dealing with why our immune systems are going wonky. How we deal with our exercise, how we deal with stress, and of eating human food.

Elle: I know you've seen it, where someone's antibodies were 700, they adopt a paleo lifestyle, and then their antibodies go down below

100. I guess the big message for Hashimoto's patients is: You can be optimized on thyroid hormone replacement as a Hashimoto's patient, but if your doctor doesn't care about your levels of antibodies, you are with the wrong doctor! Because that doctor has no idea that you can even do anything about the levels of antibodies—they just don't know it's possible. If doctors just knew about the grain component to Hashimoto's and were very serious about impressing it upon their patients, their patients would have lower and lower levels of antibodies and less risk of developing other immune issues, cancers, etc.

Dr. Foresman: Correct. And that improvement is enormous for long-term health. Of course, you're saying, "Correcting the thyroid hormone appropriately is imperative, but you can correct that while still having a whole crap-load of dysfunction," meaning you're still autoimmune. We have to make people aware that they are missing the point if all they look at is thyroid hormone replacement. We really have to correct this autoimmune dysfunction. That's why this is so important that the focus isn't just on the appropriate thyroid hormone (which it is, of course), but it's on correcting the underlying problem. That's why, especially when you emphasize the paleo/primal approach, that's really correcting the underlying cause, which is *autoimmune thyroid*. That is, for the long-term, going to make such a huge difference in people's health, rather than just focusing on whether they have the right T3 and Reverse T3 levels, etc.

Elle: We discussed two antibody tests earlier for Hashimoto's. What kind of levels of antibodies are you looking for to be *optimal*?

Dr. Foresman: To be quite honest with you, even if they are within reference range in all these labs, that's still measuring cross-reacting antibodies. So you should be unmeasurable on most of those tests. That should be your goal, period.

Elle: Wait, as in the antibodies aren't even there?

Dr. Foresman: Right. As if they don't have them. That is the goal, to not have any, and it's achievable.

Elle: So you're saying that someone with Hashimoto's who is optimized on thyroid hormone replacement can actually get to the point where it doesn't even look like they have Hashimoto's on lab results?

Dr. Foresman: Absolutely.

Elle: Wow! That *is* optimal. That's amazing. I didn't know you could get them down to *undetectable* status.

Dr. Foresman: That's what you're looking for, is *unmeasurable* thyroglobulin antibodies and thyroid peroxidase antibodies. That should be your goal. I mean, if they start with a level greater than 3,000 and they end up at 100, you have done so much benefit for them. And then whatever it is that can make them never go away completely, I don't want people worrying about that. But in the end, you really do want to shoot for unmeasurable levels of thyroid antibodies, TPO and Tg antibodies.

Elle: Other than grains that exacerbate the antibody situation, I'm assuming that other factors like general inflammation from food or other things, is that also part of the immunity scenario, or it's really just grains that trigger it?

Dr. Foresman: It's the grains. But the key is, as you know, a main component is healing the gut, right? It goes back to healing the gut first, making sure you deal with leaky gut, healthy gastrointestinal flora. People who have other chronic viruses, they tend to have problems getting their antibody levels down, so dealing with other forms of viral infections, dealing with leaky gut, dealing with gastrointestinal flora. It actually gets to be relatively complicated for some people, but the majority of people, it's a simple thing we've talked about; even using low-dose naltrexone is useful in helping with the autoimmune thyroid stuff.

Elle: Tell us about naltrexone.

Dr. Foresman: In treating autoimmune thyroid disease, I have found the three most vital treatments. Incorporating a paleo/primal lifestyle, combined with correcting vitamin D (levels 70–90), and providing methylselenocysteine (selenium) at 200 mcg twice daily, will usually cause thyroid antibodies to drop. If I am convinced the patient has been compliant with these recommendations, and yet antibodies are not falling appropriately, the addition of low-dose naltrexone (LDN) could help significantly. The website www.lowdosenaltrexone.org serves as a good reference. Obtained from a compounding pharmacy with a doctor's prescription, at a dose of 4.5 mg nightly, naltrexone boosts natural endorphin levels and can serve as a significant immunomodulator, helping reduce thyroid antibodies.

Paleo/Primal Resources

With internet access, living a paleo life is easy to figure out. There are a ton of paleo recipes online, and more and more paleo products are becoming available to purchase at health food stores and online. MarksDailyApple.com is an incredible resource for any questions you may have about health issues and/or primal living. There are myriad online resources—books, podcasts, online blogs—to continually educate yourself on paleo/primal living. Even though I am a Primal Blueprint Certified Expert and I coach people on this topic, I continue to listen, read, and reread what other paleo/primal authors, podcast hosts, and speakers have to say. I always learn something new, even if it's just a different perspective.

Resources for Paleo and Thyroid Health
PALEO, THYROID, AND LIFE COACHING

Elle Russ: www.elleruss.com (Paleo, Thyroid, and Life Coaching)
Jeffrey Brownstein: Shine@LifePurposeU.com (Life Coaching)
Eli Rohde: EliGirl@gmail.com (Paleo Coaching, former vegetarian)
Janie Bowthorpe: www.StopTheThyroidMadness.com
     (Thyroid Coaching)
Cassie Parks: www.cassieparks.com (Life Coaching)
Annie Botticelli: www.AnnieHelpsYou.com (Life Coaching)

BOOKS

The Primal Blueprint by Mark Sisson
Brain Maker by David Perlmutter, MD
CT3M Handbook by Paul Robinson (For people with lingering
     adrenal issues on T3-only hormone replacement.)

BOOKS cont'd

Grain Brain by David Perlmutter, MD
Habits of a Happy Brain by Loretta Graziano Breuning, PhD
Keto Clarity by Jimmy Moore with Eric C. Westman, MD
No Grain, No Pain by Dr. Peter Osborne
Paleo Girl by Leslie Klenke
Paleo Manifesto by John Durant
Recovering with T3 by Paul Robinson
Stop the Thyroid Madness by Janie A. Bowthorpe, MEd
The Perfect Human Diet by C. J. Hunt
The Wild Diet by Abel James

FILMS

The Perfect Human Diet – C. J. Hunt (Documentary and book)

FREE PODCASTS

Fat-Burning Man (Abel James)
The Livin' La Vida Low-Carb Show (Jimmy Moore)
The Primal Blueprint Podcast (Primal Blueprint)
Underground Wellness (Sean Croxton)
The Primal Endurance Podcast (For people interested in competitive
   sports and athlete-level training.)

PALEO/PRIMAL/LOW-CARB WEBSITES AND BLOGS

MarksDailyApple.com (The most comprehensive daily blog on
      primal living!)
FatBurningMan.com
LivingLaVidaLowCarb.com

ONLINE THYROID PATIENT-TO-PATIENT GROUPS

NTH (Natural Thyroid Hormones) Yahoo group
RT3-Adrenals Yahoo group

PALEO/PRIMAL RECIPES

CindysTable.com (Over eight hundred free paleo recipes!)
EasyPaleo.com
MarksDailyApple.com
PaleoGrubs.com
PaleoLeap.com
PaleoPorn.net
StupidEasyPaleo.com

Find a Paleo Doctor

PrimalDocs.com
PaleoPhysiciansNetwork.com

Websites to Do Your Own Blood Work

PrivateMDLabs.com
MyMedLab.com
DirectLabs.com

high-carbohydrate, high-insulin-producing diet, 107
ketosis, 187
T3, 95–96
thyroid hormone metabolism, 240, 248
paleo/primal lifestyle, 5, 280–282
selenium, 270
methylation, 59
methylcobalamin, 60
methylselenocysteine, 291
Midwest "Goiter Belt", 6, 69, 131
milk thistle, 83
*The Mindful Carnivore: A Vegetarian's Hunt
for Sustenance*, 128
minerals
conversion of T4 to T3, 97
iodine, 68–70
iron, 61–64
magnesium, 56–57, 169
selenium. *See* selenium
zinc, 71
Minger, Denise, 213
misdiagnoses, 2
depression/bipolar disorder, 97–98, 250
Cara's story, 225
Elle's PCOS (Polycystic Ovary Syndrome), 3, 198
Hashimoto's, 38
mistreatment, 2–3, 27–28, 238, 243, 246,
249, 256
blood pressure medication, 261
Cara's story, 225
worst-case scenario, 245
monounsaturated fats, 136–137
Moore, Jimmy, 188, 293
Morgan's success story, 220–222
MTHFR, 58–59
multi-dosing, 48, 94–95, 257–258
muscles
glycogen, 112–114, 155
lifting heavy things, 154–155
soreness, 17, 100, 168
My Med Lab website, 294
myostatin, 154
myxedema, 18

N

naltrexone, 290–291

Nature-Throid, 43, 252
Morgan's story, 221–223
NDT (Natural Desiccated Thyroid),
42–43, 242–243, 260, 277
brands, 42–43
Armour Thyroid, 252
Nature-Throid. *See* Nature-Throid
common themes in patients optimized
on NDT, 50
dosing, 42, 45–46, 257–258
frequency, 48–49
mornings of blood tests, 50
T3 dose comparison, 93
fixing Reverse T3, 83
history of, 44–45
sublingual vs. swallowing, 47
synthetic T4/T3, 44
treatment, 44
neuropathies, 114
niacinamide (B3), 60
No Grain, No Pain, 293
norepinephrine, 38, 99
Northrup, Christiane, MD, 5, 38, 99
NP Thyroid, 42
NTH (Natural Thyroid Hormones) Yahoo
group, 53, 293
nuts, 132
paleo/primal food list, 119
peanuts, 133
sources, order of healthfulness, 132

O

oil, 140. *See also* fat (dietary)
hydrogenation, 141
olive oil, 136–137
omega-6 fatty acids, 139
paleo/primal food list, 119
omega-3 fatty acids, 138–141
EPA and DHA, 139
seafood, 131
omega-6 fatty acids, 138–141
nuts, 132
optimization, 31, 42
adjusting doses for optimization,
271–273
common themes in patients optimized
on NDT and T3-only, 50–51
Elle's story, 205

TSH (Thyroid Stimulating Hormone), 7,
    29–30
    suppression, 30–35, 245–256
    testing, 23–24, 26, 32–33
TSI (thyroid-stimulating immunoglobu-
    lin), 12
tubers, 133
type 2 diabetes, 111–116, 212
    Hawaii, 211–212
    HbA1c test, 188–189
    testing, 72–73

U

underactive thyroid. *See* hypothyroidism
Underground Wellness podcast, 293
undiagnosis, 27
unhealthy patterns, 191–194

V

vaccenic acid, 141
vegans/vegetarians, 127–128
vegetable oil, 138, 141
vegetables, 123–125
    growing methods, 124
    nutritional values, 125
    paleo/primal food list, 117
    The Primal Blueprint Food Pyramid,
        116
    starchy vegetables, 133
visualization, 174–175
vitals, 29
    tracking, 76, 77
vitamins
    B12 and homocysteine (and other B
        vitamins), 57–61
    conversion of T4 to T3, 97

C, 71–72
    high-dose vitamin C for inflamma-
        tion, 190
    organic acids urine test, 191
    D, 66–68
    paleo/primal food list, 120
Volek, Jeff S., 188

W

walking, 153
Web resources for paleo/primal, 292–294
websites to do your own blood work, 294
weighing yourself, 193–194
weights, lifting heavy things, 154–155
Westman, Eric C., MD, 188, 293
whole grains, 143, 145
Why We Get Fat, 136
The Wild Diet, 293
wild rice, 117, 133
    The Primal Blueprint Food Pyramid,
        116
WP Thyroid, 43, 252

Y

Yahoo groups, 53, 293
yogurt, 133
You Can Heal Your Life, 174

Z

zinc, 71
    conversion of T4 to T3, 97

OTHER BOOKS BY **PRIMAL BLUEPRINT PUBLISHING**

MARK SISSON

 The Primal Connection

 The Primal Blueprint

 The Primal Blueprint 21-Day Total Body Transformation

 The Primal Blueprint 90-Day Journal: A Personal Experiment (n=1)

 Primal Blueprint Box Set: Includes the original "Primal Blueprint" hardcover, "The Primal Connection," "The Primal Blueprint Cookbook," "The Primal Blueprint Quick & Easy Meals," and "Primal Blueprint Healthy Sauces, Dressings & Toppings"

MARK SISSON AND BRAD KEARNS

 Primal Endurance

COOKBOOKS BY MARK SISSON AND JENNIFER MEIER

 The Primal Blueprint Cookbook

 The Primal Blueprint Quick and Easy Meals

 The Primal Blueprint Healthy Sauces, Dressings, and Toppings

OTHER AUTHORS

 The Hidden Plague by Tara Grant

 Rich Food, Poor Food by Mira Calton, CN, and Jayson Calton, Ph.D.

 Death by Food Pyramid by Denise Minger

 The South Asian Health Solution by Ronesh Sinha, MD

 Paleo Girl by Leslie Klenke

 Lil' Grok Meets the Korgs by Janée Meadows

 The Primal Prescription by Doug McGuff, MD and Robert P. Murphy, PhD

COOKBOOKS

 The Paleo Primer by Keris Marsden and Matt Whitmore

 Primal Cravings by Brandon and Megan Keatle

 Fruit Belly by Romy Dollé

 Good Fat, Bad Fat by Romy Dollé